Just Grow It Yourself

Home Gardens Outshine
Industrial Food

David G. Fisher

Just Grow It Yourself

Quantity sales special discounts are available on quantity purchases by corporations, associations, and others. For details, contact the publisher at the address above.

Orders by U.S. trade bookstores and wholesalers. Email info@ BeyondPublishing.net

The Beyond Publishing Speakers Bureau can bring authors to your live event. For more information or to book an event contact the Beyond Publishing Speakers Bureau speak@BeyondPublishing.net

The Author can be reached directly at JustGrowItYourself.com

Manufactured and printed in the United States of America distributed globally by BeyondPublishing.net

BEYOND
PUBLISHING

New York | Los Angeles | London | Sydney

ISBN: 978-1-637926-90-1

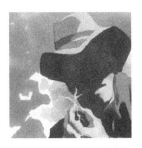

Dedicated to my dad, a prodigious gardener

who inspires me to this day.

Contents

1

A Food Interview
with America

Good morning, America! How are you this bright and cheerful day?

"Bright and cheerful? Maybe for some. Frankly, I'm not exactly feeling like a million bucks, which I think has a lot to do with what I eat. And speaking of millions, I see these marvelous supermarkets all over my country brimming with food, yet pre-COVID-19, 49 million of my people didn't have enough to eat, which experts say has increased by at least 17 million with the pandemic. Even before the virus, five million of my children were too small and thin for their age—right here in one of the world's richest countries. I thought stunting was something you only see in desperately poor countries.

But how can that be? We have plenty of food, at least twice as much as we need to feed everyone.

"I don't know where it all goes, but that brings up an even bigger problem: eating too much. Of my 331 million citizens, 231 million are overweight, of which 132 million are obese. Even 8 million of my children are now obese, and it starts at age two. All of which has led to some 165 million—nearly half my population—to being diabetic or pre-diabetic. I have an epidemic on top of a pandemic."

Mercy! I can see why you're not feeling cheerful.

"Meanwhile, modern farming loses two billion tons of my topsoil every year, at ten times the rate it's being replaced.[1] How on earth am I supposed to grow food when it's gone?

My food companies spend $11 billion peddling junk food each year, often targeting the most vulnerable of my people—children and the poor.

Over $1 trillion of the health, social, and environmental costs of food production don't show up in the prices my people pay at the grocery store.

As if all that's not enough, wasted food costs my economy $2.6 trillion a year.[2]

And on and on it goes in the dreadful millions, billions, and trillions of dollars. I'm truly a mess of 'ill'-ions.

So yeah, I'm hanging in there, but I sure could stand to be a lot less ill. Which is to say, I'm seriously hurting."

This poignant, imaginary interview with our beloved country highlights my reason for writing this book: to address our food-derived hurting in the millions, billions, and trillions by much more fully engaging a powerful, effective solution that so far has been almost completely overlooked—home gardens. First, I want to inspire potential new gardeners, as well as those currently gardening to expand their efforts. Second, I'd like to motivate policymakers and community leaders to leverage individual efforts enormously. Gardeners are on the front lines, and policymakers are the strategic support teams. They need each other, and each should be aware of everything that's primarily directed to the other to make the most of their own role.

Why turn to home gardens? To begin with, the industrial food system is failing. It's unsustainable in the long term and struggling even in the short run, especially with getting food to the low-income. COVID-19 has made the system's shortcomings all the more obvious, and it appears that this pandemic is going to be with us awhile. Although advocates of sustainable/regenerative agriculture have promoted many worthwhile solutions to food production and distribution, they've missed the vast potential of home gardens. These gardens, contrary to the common narrative, are not only an extraordinarily potent source of food production, they're much more efficient, with far greater returns for the energy and effort, than industrial food.

All of which adds up to my primary proposal: a three-tiered food system, anchored by 1) home gardens, backed up by

2) local food production, in turn complemented by 3) pared-down distant food production, that could plausibly replace much to most industrially produced food. This system would save trillions in costs to human health, the economy, and the environment. It would not replace non-food use of crops for purely industrial purposes, such as corn and soybeans for fuel. My secondary assertion is that food gardens can be the most promising and dignified path to permanent food accessibility not just for those who are better off, but also, and especially for those who are less well-off. Don't believe it? Then read on: I'll show you why it's genuinely workable. We'll begin with the example of victory gardens.

2

The Good News:
It's Been Done Before

Victory Gardens, Just What Are They?

I've been surprised—perhaps even shocked—by the number of younger Americans who've never heard of victory gardens. Coined by the great agricultural scientist, George Washington Carver, this term of ringing hope designated home vegetable gardens that supplemented food production during times of war. Victory gardens in World War II were common not only in the United States but also in Canada, Australia, and Great Britain. At a perilous time, when the U.S. was feeding its own civilian and military populations as well as helping to supply those of its allies, these emblems of patriotic optimism numbered 20 million in the U.S. alone. It was a serious business, as U-boats were sinking hundreds of food-laden ships headed for Britain. As you might expect, civilians stepped up and loyally answered the government's call to action. According to the USDA, at their peak in 1944 victory gardens accounted for 40 percent of the nation's vegetable production.

People used every available spot to grow at least something, no matter how seemingly insignificant. "Small things count" was the mantra. Vegetables

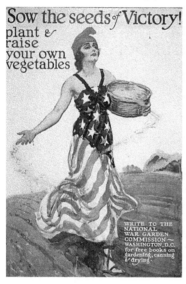

sprouted from yards and vacant lots, as well as containers on rooftops, patios, porches, and even on fire escapes. Appeals to patriotism appeared in every form, including what amounted to sex appeal, to get people going. Doing its share, the venerable magazine *Life* ran gardening come-ons featuring "pretty girls in becoming shorts".

The value of those gardens was $1.2 billion, or $17.2 billion in today's dollars. Unfortunately, once the war was over, and especially as the production of wartime explosives and nerve gas transformed into the chemical fertilizers and pesticides of industrial agriculture, many people gave up on their victory gardens.

But not everyone. I remember boyhood visits to my grandmother, who lived in Roanoke Rapids in eastern North Carolina. She always had a few rows of butterbeans, tomatoes, and sweet peppers out back, as did her next-door neighbor "Miz Edwards" and others nearby. I grew up thinking that backyard gardens were normal for residential areas of small towns, even though it was years after the war was over.

I lived in the countryside of the mountains, in the western part of the state. When I was just a toddler my dad had a large garden, but the pressures of doubling the size of our house plus a full-time job soon forced him to give it up. Then, when I was about twelve years old, I launched my first vegetable garden, starting with a hand-spaded 4' x 8' plot. That garden became my pride and joy, and I enlarged it with each succeeding summer. By the time I graduated from high school and went off to college, it measured about 80' x 100', lush with corn, beans, tomatoes, green peppers, potatoes, spinach, mustard greens, squash, and more.

Over the ensuing decades, I grew a garden whenever I could—in Virginia, Wisconsin, and now Iowa, where I've had one for about ten years. My most recent garden, in 2020, was only 27' x 31', but I got a lot of produce out of that plot, as you'll see presently.

What's a garden worth?

There are a number of ways to measure the value of a food garden: cash profit, total weight of the produce, yield (weight per unit area), survival value (how long you could survive on your garden produce alone), and intangibles such as exercise, exposure to sunshine and fresh air, and communing with nature. These measures are usually tied together, but since most people are money-oriented, especially in this time of high unemployment, that's a good place to start.

Cash profit

Here you will see three very different approaches to assessing cash value: a family of four eating almost entirely from their garden for a year, my own experience with red heirloom corn in my 2019 garden, and an online service that automatically computes the planning for a 15' x 20' vegetable garden.

Perhaps the most comprehensive and insightful of these, at least on a family scale, is the first. That's what Barbara Kingsolver—the novelist—and her family did for a year back in about 2004. To me, their experience came across as the ultimate example of family food security and empowerment. That is, short of holing up in an underground bunker with a year's supply of preserved food and water in some remote corner of Montana.

Meticulously chronicled in her book, *Animal, Vegetable, Miracle—A Year of Food Life*, her goal was to see if a "normal-ish" American family in Virginia could be content on the fruits of their local foodshed for a year. That meant raising and eating their own chickens and turkeys, as well as a variety of vegetables, all on their own land. The youngest girl separately raised chickens for eggs, further integrating food choices with self-sufficiency. They allowed a few edibles to come from off-farm, as long as they were locally produced and in season. That meant no oranges, chocolate, almonds, raisins, or almost anything else that had to be produced thousands of miles away and shipped in by environmentally costly, petroleum-fed ships and trucks.

They did grant themselves one luxury item each, in limited quantities, on the condition that they'd learn how to purchase it through a channel most beneficial to the grower and the land where it grew. That let in coffee, dried fruit, hot chocolate, and a few spices such as cinnamon and cloves. I think they also allowed non-local flour and oatmeal, although the book isn't entirely clear on that point.

In any case, they were able to accomplish it, partly as a result of careful planning over the previous several years, including trying it out on a more modest, test garden a year in advance. As you can imagine, many surprises popped up. A pleasant one was that it brought them closer together as a family. But there were also some significant challenges, as with just about any garden.

Nevertheless, between April and November the full cash value of the vegetables, chickens, and turkeys they raised and harvested was $4,410, or $6,018 today, adjusted for inflation. To get that figure they assigned a price to the fruits, vegetables, and poultry per pound on the basis of organic products on the market at that time.

Altogether, it gives you an indication of what's possible. And the reason that it's more appropriate to consider organic than conventional food is that organic is closer to what most people would do at home. Conventional food is cheaper at the checkout counter, but that's only because it doesn't include the "externalized" economic, social, environmental, and health costs of industrial agriculture. More on that later. Meanwhile, organic uses more natural methods that avoid many of those negative costs, resulting in higher but more honest prices.

Some will surely protest: "A Kingsolver-type deal is way too ambitious for me. Can't I do something that's a little more realistic?" Sure. So next, consider the second case study of garden evaluation: the section of my little garden where I grew four 22' rows of corn in 2019.

Corn is perhaps the most iconic of American crops. It will grow almost anywhere—some varieties even in Alaska—but it's especially dominant in the Midwest and Great Plains. It can produce very high yields and can be used fresh or in dried products like cornmeal and grits, as well as in a wide variety of ultra-processed forms like high-fructose corn syrup and chicken nuggets. However, the corn that's consumed directly by humans is only a small fraction of the truly enormous U.S. output (14.2 billion bushels in 2018-19). Over 90 percent of it goes to fuel, livestock feed, and a host of non-food industrial products dispersed throughout our culture. Truth be told, it's more comprehensively American than apple pie. By far.

Besides all that, it's my favorite vegetable (technically, it's a grain), and not just because of its fabulous taste freshly boiled on the cob and dripping with salted butter, or as heirloom breakfast grits with scrambled eggs and sausage. It's also because there's just something personal and magical about the plants themselves. I get such an inspiring lift from walking amongst them in my garden, their broad, green, friendly leaves spread out like welcoming arms. Maybe that's why corn was so central to the Aztecs, Incas, Mayans, and other Mesoamerican cultures. So it seems entirely appropriate to use corn as another example of the kind of return you can get from a very modest outlay in seeds and effort.

In 2019 I planted and harvested 36 pounds of dry, shelled kernels from a 16' x 22' plot of heirloom red corn. Interestingly, this is remarkably close to the 35.2 pounds of corn products the average person consumed in 2018,

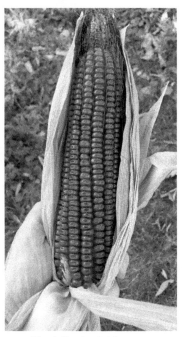

Bloody Butcher heirloom corn

according to the USDA.[1] The nearest market match for my grits is made from the same variety of corn that I used—"Bloody Butcher" (I would have chosen a different name for it). But, it isn't organic and would cost me $13.97 per pound as of this writing. The closest match for my cornmeal is a whole-grain brand of organic cornmeal at $9.92 per pound. Since my grinding and sifting process yields grits and cornmeal at a ratio of 2:1 (24 to 12 pounds, respectively), my grits are currently worth $335.28 and my cornmeal $119.04, for a grand harvest total of $454.32. Not bad for a $4 investment of seed corn and a little care and cultivation. (For those who want to see the calculations in detail, on these as well as other figures I cite, see Appendices 1 and 2.)

But to play the garden devil's advocate (and there *is* a garden devil who will strike sooner or later, as any long-time gardener will tell you), why not just buy regular, cheap grits at the grocery store? Well for starters, you'd be getting a significantly deficient product. According to the USDA, cornmeal made from a similar heirloom variety of red corn (Floriani Red Flint) has 60 percent more nutritional value—in ten essential nutrients including protein, fiber, vitamins, and minerals—than cornmeal made from conventional corn[2]. That's because corn meant for conventional production, like most other industrially-produced fruits and vegetables, is typically grown in nutritionally-deficient soil, hence the need for heavy chemical fertilizer applications. It has also been bred over the last 70 years for traits like appearance, shipping toughness, and shelf life, rather than nutrition.

Continuing to play the adversarial angle, why not just buy very similar matches for my grits and cornmeal, which you can easily get online? After all, they would be pesticide- and GMO-free, and would likely have the same enhanced flavor and nutrition that mine do. I'd say, sure, go ahead—if you don't mind shelling out about $450 for something you can get for an initial seed investment of $4.

Of course, this assumes that you go about your gardening enterprise sensibly, not killing yourself with an over-ambitious ramping up of intense physical work you're not used to. Start small, and increase gradually. You have to make it a fun, comfortable, and enjoyable ride if you want to reap the full benefits of a home garden.

The third example of evaluating the profitability of growing your own veggies is to use an online gardening service, of which there are many, such as Born to Grow (borntogrow.net). Basically, the service employs apps and website gardening calendars to take much of the guesswork out of knowing when, where, and how to plan and grow a vegetable garden. To illustrate with one of its simpler examples (as of 2020), it said that by using its plug-and-play garden plan you can grow $1,000 worth of vegetables on 300 square feet of garden space—a 15' x 20' plot—over six months.

When I first saw that claim I was doubtful. $1,000 is more than twice the value I got from my 352 square foot corn plot, which was 17 percent larger than their plot. However, I noticed that they packed their plot of 20 vegetables and herbs pretty tight, with aisles only a foot wide, whereas my corn was generously spaced at 4 feet between the rows, and with aisles 2 feet wide. Hmm ... Could I be a little more efficient?

So I did the math and found that if I converted to the standard, recommended spacing for corn—2.5 feet between rows and 6 inches between plants in a row—then with six rows, 20 feet long (same size plot as Born to Grow's), I'd have 240 plants, as opposed to the 100 I grew in my larger plot. I don't think the closer spacing would reduce yield, as I noticed that even where my plants were only four to five inches apart the stalks were just as robust, and the ears every bit as large and well filled out as with stalks eight to ten inches apart. (The spacing within the rows averaged 10.5 inches.) In any case, it's what is used commercially, which is intended to get the highest yields possible.

At the 0.36 pounds of corn per plant[i] that I got for my 2019 plot, and using the closest match in market price that I could find for my grits and cornmeal, I found that with standard spacing, I would get a total value of $1,071 for a 15' x 20' plot of my red heirloom corn. And that doesn't take into account Born to Grow's successive planting of more than one vegetable in a given space over six months. By contrast, I would grow only corn on a 300 square foot plot, and for only four months. Nor did their plan take into account the estimated $70 cost of seed packets for 20 vegetables and herbs in their garden. Versus my revised plan using reduced spacing and more plants, which would cost me only $8 for two packets of seed corn. So yeah, based on my experience with heirloom corn, producing $1,000 worth of vegetables and herbs over six months on a 15' x 20' plot—given a little basic gardening knowledge—is quite reasonable. I'd say if the online approach appeals to you, then go for it.

In addition to these examples, here are summaries of a few other cost/benefit analyses for home garden scenarios I scrounged from the Internet:

- After spending $2.5 billion on seeds, supplies, and other upfront costs in 2008, American gardeners reaped a $21

---

i   The dried kernels of an individual ear of corn can add up to 0.7 lb. or more, which, since each plant typically has only one ear, would be 0.7 lb. per stalk. This applies to both heirloom and commercial corn.

billion return on their investment. For the average 600 square foot garden, that comes out to a profit of about $530.[3]

- On average, home vegetable gardens produce $677 worth of fruits and vegetables beyond the $238 cost of materials and supplies.[4]

- Every $1 invested in a garden yields $6 worth of fresh produce. Some vegetables yield even better returns. $1 spent growing green beans gets you produce valued at $75.[5]

- For investing $70 in seeds and supplies you could grow 350 pounds of vegetables worth about $600. So, you would save, for an average 600 square foot garden, over $500.[6]

- As an example of an individual case study, in 2009, Roger and Jacqueline Dorion calculated the worth of their 4,000 square foot garden by keeping track of costs, then weighing everything they grew and noting the price at three markets: a local grocery store, a farmer's market, and Whole Foods. Their garden netted them $2,431, or the equivalent of $3,026 today.[7]

Bear in mind that most of the costs in these examples are likely one-time, up-front expenses. Once you've invested in hand tools, fencing, a garden hose, and maybe a wheelbarrow, you don't need to buy them again, as they become a fixed cost that can be amortized over many years. I certainly don't have to spend $238 or even $70 worth of materials and supplies every year; it's more like $15 to $20 for new seeds (when I grow my own starter plants), seed potatoes, and sweet potato starter slips.

Total harvest weight

This measure has limited value, because, by itself, it doesn't indicate what proportion of your harvest is simply water. If your garden has a lot of tomatoes, watermelons, cucumbers, zucchinis, cabbages, and the like, you'll have impressive amounts of weight, but 80 percent or more of it will be water. The same weight in dried corn or beans will have much more energy and nutritional value. So, when someone tells me they grew 600 pounds of produce in their garden, I say "Great. What all did you grow?" Weight, alone, just doesn't tell me much.

Yield (harvest per unit area)

Yield is how much harvest you get per square foot or acre, whether the harvest is measured in volume—such as bushels— or weight. But like weight alone, yield can sound much more impressive if most of your produce is watery, bulky vegetables than if it's lightweight items that are more nutrient- or calorie-dense.

Survival value

By this I mean that if you were to rely on just your garden, how many months would it feed you while maintaining good health? In order to keep you alive and robust until harvest time the following year, you'd need to grow the right ratio of calorie-rich vegetables like corn and potatoes (which are also nutritious, by the way) to those like tomatoes and greens that are low in calories but rich in other kinds of nutrients. That's why if you tell me you can stay healthy for a year eating only from your garden, it's much more meaningful than measures of weight or yield. For some, it may even be the best way to ensure access to reliable, healthy food, as we'll see in the next chapter.

Various garden plans predict how large your garden should be per individual or family to meet most or all of their food needs for a year. It depends on many factors, so an average figure doesn't mean much. Suffice it to say that they range, per person, from a low of 500 square feet with intensive Permaculture[8] to 4,000 square feet at intermediate yields of biointensive[9], to a high of maybe 6,000 square feet.

As for my corn, I'm from the south and love grits, so I let it dry on the stalks, then harvest, grind it up with a hand-cranked grain meal, and sift it with a kitchen strainer and sieve to produce grits as well as cornmeal. The grinding and sifting only takes about five minutes per serving of grits, so it's a snap, and satisfying to prepare. Because these products are produced fresh-on-the-spot from whole-kernel corn, they taste far more genuinely corn-savory than the highly processed, bland grits you get in grocery stores and restaurants. Plus, I get considerably more nutrition, as you saw with the heirloom red corn compared with conventional corn. That's partly because processing removes the hull and germ, which is where a good bit of the nutrition is.

Intangibles

Other things you miss out on if you just buy all your food at the supermarket are better taste, increased exercise, and exposure to the sun, fresh air, garden plants, and the earth. Not to mention the joy, satisfaction, and feeling of empowerment that comes from growing and eating your own food. And don't forget the added food security—possibly the most important of all in these uncertain times. Even, surprisingly, for some who are relatively well-off.

What's the total monetary value of all those extras? Hard to say, but if you could "dollarize" the lifetime health benefits that would result from growing the corn yourself, it would likely much more than make up for any cost "savings" derived from cheap food. Not that we need to cast all of life's values in terms of dollars. We certainly don't, but it is the most common measure used.

Maybe, just growing what you enjoy tending, harvesting, and eating, according to the energy, resources, and time you're willing to put into it, is enough. If you truly enjoy gardening, the added benefits can make it all worthwhile, even if it only supplements what you get elsewhere. A Princeton study found that home gardening ranked among the top five out of fifteen activities that produce emotional well-being, including frequency of experiencing peak positive emotions, and that vegetable gardening outranked growing flowers.[10]

As you can see, there are a variety of ways to gauge the value of a vegetable garden. I'll go into more on planning and growing later, but the Kingsolvers' experience, my corn plot, and Born to Grow give you an idea of real dollar value.

Now, to illustrate how different aspects of cash value, yield, weight, survival value, and intangibles can come together, I'd like to talk a little more about my corn, which contributes to the evidence that home gardens are far more efficient and economical than the industrial food system.

Home garden vs. conventional corn

It's not just the basics—the 86.4 pounds of corn I could get from a 15' x 20' plot, or the $1,071 value thereof, or even all the other positives mentioned so far—it's the practical results that count. That amount of corn, if converted entirely into highly nutritious, whole-grain grits, would provide 917 generous, 1.5 oz. servings (cooked, 6.5 oz. each). Enough to grace the breakfast of one person every day for two-and-a-half years, or of two people for a year and three months.

Don't like grits? Or worse, don't even know what grits are? It's okay, I'll forgive you—this time—if you're not from the South. So fine, grind the corn down into 86.4 pounds of equally nutritious cornmeal—for cornbread, corn dumplings, hoecakes (another traditional Southern favorite), breading, or other culinary corn delights. That would probably also last two people for at least a year.

So how does that compare with commercial corn yield? Well, matching my results of 0.36 pounds of corn per stalk and the 86.4 pounds of corn that I could grow in a 300 square foot plot, the harvest would be 1.42 bushels. That works out to a yield rate of 226 bushels per acre, compared to 168 bushels per acre for the 2019 U.S. average yield for corn.

Or, consider the all-important angle of nitrogen fertilizer. Industrial corn is said to require about one pound of applied nitrogen for every bushel of corn produced. Since the U.S. yield of corn for 2018-19 was 168 bushels per acre, that presumably required an average of at least 168 pounds of nitrogen per acre. The Penn State University Extension Service recommends a little more, 220 pounds of nitrogen fertilizer per acre, to get a yield of 200 bu. of corn per acre. Yet under the conditions I prescribed, I'd get a yield rate of 226 bushels per acre with an application rate of only 83 pounds of (organic) nitrogen per acre. So, I'd get a 35 percent higher rate of yield (226/168) using only 38 percent of Penn State's recommended use of nitrogen fertilizer per acre (83/220).

Now, what if everyone (who has a sunny space and could) grew their own corn? How would it compare to the truly gargantuan U.S. corn industry?

That calls for considering how backyard gardens could add up. There are about 102 million American homes that have lawns, the average size of which is about 10,000 square feet. Meaning, it's very likely that most of those lawns could accommodate a 300 square foot garden. If a little corn plot of that size—with standard plant spacing—was tucked into a corner of each of those lawns, and the yield per stalk equaled mine, the total yield would be 144 million bushels. That's slightly more than 1% of the 14 billion bushels that the U.S. averaged in corn production over 2018-2019. And since much less than

10 percent of the national yield goes to actually feeding people directly (including high-fructose corn syrup and all the corn in junk foods), well ... do you begin to get the picture? Even if not everyone who has a lawn chose to have a food garden?

Not that we'd want backyard gardens to replace all industrially-produced corn. Presumably, almost all of it would still be needed for livestock feed and non-food purposes, of which there are many. But you can certainly see that the industry's narrative of being all-big and powerful, while your little garden plot is maybe cute but puny by comparison, inherently unable to compete with the mighty industrial machine, is grossly misleading. Besides, this analysis was just for corn. As you will see later, you can get equally impressive results with other home-grown vegetables, compared to industrial production.

Victory Gardens: 1944 and Today

To get back to victory gardens, the relative numbers of households growing their own vegetables provide yet another way of gauging the potential value of home food gardens:

1944

- There were 20 million food gardens in the U.S. population of about 132 million, which means that the number of gardens per capita was 0.15, or, rounded off, one garden for about every seven people.

- Nevertheless, those gardens provided 40 percent of all U.S. consumed vegetables at that time, according to the USDA.

2019-20

- In 2019, there were 43 million household food gardens in a population of about 331 million, which means that there were 0.13 gardens per capita, not a big difference from the ratio of 0.15 for 1944.

- But what percentage of all U.S. vegetables consumed now are grown in home gardens? Unknown. I contacted the USDA, and they said they don't keep such records now. Nor does the National Gardening Association, which has a plethora of other home food gardening statistics.

However, today's gardeners may contribute a good bit less toward a well-fortified subsistence diet than their counterparts did in 1945. At that time, the authors of the 1943 USDA *Victory Garden Leader's Handbook* were well aware that—especially in wartime—people needed energy as well as vitamins and minerals. So, they recommended the following consumption of vegetables in pounds per week per person:

• Leafy green and yellow vegetables	3.5
• Tomatoes and cabbage	2.0
Total	5.5
• Corn, beets, parsnips, turnips, etc.	3.0
• White and sweet potatoes	3.5
• Dried peas and beans	3.5
Total	10.0

In other words, they urged people to eat almost twice as much calorie-rich vegetables as low-calorie veggies. They also urged victory gardeners to plan out how much of each item to plant, so as to harvest and store enough to tide their families over until the following year's garden started to produce.

By contrast, today's gardeners, ranked by the percentages who grow various vegetables, are listed below.[11] The vegetables they favor are almost all in the category of nutritious but watery and calorie-poor:

- Tomatoes—86%
- Cucumbers—47%
- Sweet peppers—46%
- Green beans—39%
- Carrots—34%
- Summer squash—32%
- Onions—32%
- Hot peppers—31%
- Lettuce—28%
- Peas—24%
- Sweet corn—23%

Of the most calorie-rich staples (corn, dry beans, winter squash, and regular and sweet potatoes), only corn makes it into the top ten, and then just barely. Today's gardeners love their gardens and enjoy fresh produce while saving money, but they raise few calorie-rich staples. In addition, their main reason to garden is more to improve taste than to attain a significant degree of self-sufficiency.

We're not in a large-scale war, but as noted in Chapter 1, the number of Americans without enough to eat has risen from 49 million in 2019 to at least 66 million (as we'll see shortly), and probably many more as of March 2021. Given the ongoing challenges wrought by the pandemic, today's home food gardeners would be well-advised to grow significant amounts of both calorie-rich and low-calorie vegetables (bearing in mind that they're all nutrient-rich), and when feasible, to share their bounty. If they did, they could provide much to most of what the nation needs in vegetables, at a far lower total cost than that incurred by the industrial food system.

After all, the number of gardens per capita today is almost as high as it was during wartime victory gardens, so the gardening infrastructure is already in place. If we ramped up the numbers of gardeners and overall production while increasing the proportion of staples, it should be relatively easy to reach not only 40 percent of needed vegetable production but well beyond it, in short order.

Still not convinced? Consider this: Nigeria grows 50 percent of the vegetables its people eat in home gardens on just 2 percent of its cropland, and Cuba grows 60 percent of its vegetables on small urban plots.[12] So why shouldn't American gardeners, with all the resource advantages we have over those countries, be able to match their home garden food-growing capacity— or even do much better?

No matter how you look at it—from various cost/benefit analyses, to my actual and potential home garden yield rates compared to those of the industrial food system, to 1944 victory gardens vs. what 2021 victory gardens could do, to potential U.S. home garden output compared with that in Nigeria and Cuba, and especially when you consider all those factors together— what you can do with a vegetable garden is *powerful*.

3

Why Victory Gardens Now?

A gardener's warning

True, we're not in another world war. But we do have a pretty serious pandemic, which sometimes feels like a war, and it will likely still be lurching along by the time this book is published. Prescient here is the title of Steve Solomon's *Gardening When It Counts*, published in 2005, and especially its subtitle: *Growing Food in Hard Times*.

Hard times in 2005? What hard times? Turns out he was predicting events that would make growing your own veggie garden a good idea, though most people didn't pay much attention. Until now. Compare his warnings with what's happened:

- 2005: With the decline of oil will come an increase in the cost of everything made from oil: fuel for transportation, food, clothing, plastics, housing, etc.

- 2020: The great energy transition, from fossil and nuclear to sustainable renewables like wind and solar, is well underway, with roughly half the oil industry now re-orienting itself in that direction. And yes, costs have increased by 36% since 2005. But see the next comparison.

- 2005: As a result of competition with lower-cost labor and production in China and other rapidly developing countries, people in the U.S. will have less real purchasing power.

- 2020: Adding to inflation, wage stagnation and grossly increasing income disparity have reduced purchasing power for middle- and lower-income people much more than for those in high-income brackets. Meanwhile, the GDP of China, now the manufacturing hub of the world, has increased much faster than that of the U.S.

- 2005: Water supplies will decrease in many places, and watersheds will become more degraded, so water will cost more also.

- 2020: Water is a massive and varied topic that's beyond the scope of this book to adequately explore. But any water resources database or college environmental textbook will corroborate this prediction overall.

- 2005: Chemical fertilizer, especially nitrogen, is made from oil, so it also will increase in price, providing a solid reason to switch to easily-produced compost to boost soil nutrition.

- 2020: Actually, most nitrogen fertilizer is made directly from natural gas, although other fossil fuels are used to power its production. The cost of fertilizer did increase after 2005, but then it went down sharply after the 2008 recession, and has been highly variable since then. The good news is that organic fertilizers—the healthy replacement for the synthetic chemical kind—are even more widely available now than they were in 2005. Good quality compost is also much more available (though less so in urban areas) due to the huge increase in demand for organic food over the last 16 years.

So, most of Solomon's predictions have come true, making the case for starting a garden even stronger than it was in 2004. But we now also have the far more challenging COVID-19 pandemic and its continuing economic fallout to deal with. In mid-May, 2020, farmers let millions of pounds of food rot in fields and poured thousands of gallons of milk on the ground because they couldn't get those products to market. As well, they euthanized millions of unusable chickens and hogs. Yet food banks and pantries around the country were barely able to keep their shelves stocked as the newly unemployed reached out for food assistance. That situation was even more desperate in December.

And it wasn't just in the lowest-income areas. May 2020 found lines of cars a mile long at Egg Harbor food banks in New Jersey, the second-wealthiest per capita state in the U.S. To be sure, at least some of the food previously destined for schools, restaurants, hotels, cruise ships and the like was re-routed to food banks through the USDA. Yet according to a representative of the Dairy Farmers of America, the quarter of a million gallons of milk so diverted were "just a drop in the bucket."[1] There was a disjoint between excess supply and dire need, even as farmers said their losses far exceeded what the USDA was rerouting to the needy.

Even when food is available, many simply can't afford to buy it. Kate Lombardo, with the Food Bank of Lower Fairfield County in Stamford, Connecticut said, "Most people don't have that extra $100 to $200 to spend on food to ready their household for two weeks' worth of groceries."[2] Case in point: by November 2020, a quarter of the full-time population in Cape Cod, MA was food insecure.

"It's just a terrible time for a lot of people," said Catherine D'Amato, president of the Greater Boston Food Bank, the largest hunger-relief organization in New England, which provides food to 190 towns and cities in Eastern Massachusetts. "We're obviously in a crisis."[3]

Yes, the first and second economic stimulus checks helped a little, and as of this writing a third is on the way. But as *The Atlantic* put it, "If and when federal intervention dries up, millions of families just keeping their head above water will sink, as lost jobs and canceled hours force them to stop paying their rent and go into arrears on their debt payments. Hunger, homelessness, forgotten plans to attend community college, babies growing up in stressed households: these are the stakes."[4]

Meanwhile, 23.5 million Americans lack access to fresh produce, either due to high prices or because there are no grocery stores in their neighborhood.[5]

There is also a shortage of grocery store checkout clerks. Some 5,500 had contracted the corona virus by May, 100 of whom died,[6] prompting others to quit their jobs, and all to be fearful. In Iowa, Governor Reynolds even warned—contrary to state law—that food workers would lose unemployment benefits if they refused to return to a suspect workplace. A number of meat-packing plants closed as workers contracted the virus because of crowded conditions and lack of adequate safety measures. Problems caused by food worker shortages, SNAP cuts, and trade deals further undermined food availability.

The industrial food system insists that there is plenty of food, including hundreds of millions of pounds of meat in cold storage, and that the supply chain is intact, working, and resilient. But that's true only if you ignore the one in six Americans who are food insecure, and that at least a third of all food production is wasted. In addition, grocery stores, which have only a three-day supply of food at any given time, are stocked to be replaced on a steady, just-in-time basis. Whereas COVID-19 has caused pulses of panic buying, clearing out entire banks of shelves of some items, which alarms shoppers, who then engage in more panic buying. That has caused demand for staples to go up and prices to increase 10-20%, further straining the system, which was not designed for sporadic panic shopping.

The situation is in such flux it's not possible to tell whether the current food supply system can recover enough to deal effectively with the reduction in food workers, panic buying, supply chain disruptions, and food pantry shortages, especially when the full, true cost of food production is considered (see Chapter 4). What is predictable is that a large scale-up of home vegetable gardens would provide a much-needed reserve for everyone to breathe a little easier.

So indeed these are hard times, even more so than Solomon envisioned when you consider the numbers of Americans facing chronic hunger.

How can growing your own food lead us to a much better situation? Let us count the ways ...

Home gardens would:

Provide genuine food security for the low-income

This is about low-income people not getting enough of the right kinds of food to eat: under nutrition (not enough calories), malnutrition (not enough vitamins and minerals), and over nutrition (too many calories, leading to overweight and obesity). Ironically, over nutrition can be accompanied by malnutrition. That is, you can be overweight while still not getting enough vitamins, fiber, and minerals. In any case, all three forms of nutritional lack heavily impact our national life.

The USDA's most recent *Hunger Report*, published in September 2020,[7] estimated that 10.5% of the population, or 49 million people, were food-insecure in the United States. Feeding America, a nationwide network of more than two hundred food banks, predicted an additional 17 million will have trouble feeding themselves and their families as a result of the pandemic.[8] And the Institute for Research Policy at Northwestern University reported that as of June 2020, about a fourth (83 million) of the population overall, and a third of families with children, were experiencing food insecurity.[9] This translates into scenes like that in Miami, where one-and-a-half mile long lines of cars waited their turn at food banks providing 2.5 million meals a week.[10] Even with that kind of relief, the Northwestern report found that less than 10% of those facing shortages were getting access to food pantries. Let's see what this looks like at a more intimate level, down on the street.

On April 1, 2020, the *New York Times* ran a story about the only fresh grocery store in the Lower Ninth Ward of New Orleans that poignantly illustrates the plight of those who don't have reliable access to a sufficient quantity of affordable, nutritious food. The store owner and article author, Burnell Cotlon, describes the desperation of his regular customers, who were struggling with the realities of the pandemic. Everyone was scared of touching someone else. At least half of them had lost their jobs. Apologizing, they pushed food stamps, quarters, and dimes across the counter with a plastic spoon. Bartered over a 70-cent can of beans.

He cut his price for two pieces of fried chicken from $1.25 to a dollar. Watched as some people, cursing, punched their numbers again and again into the ATM machine. They had no savings, no fallback. He caught one lady shoplifting a carton of eggs, wieners, and candy bars, but let her go when she cried and said her family had nothing to eat; her man had lost his job, and they had nowhere to go. He started letting people have things on credit. His store, with 62 tabs, soon became a food pantry.

This is the kind of story—occasionally described in passing for other destitute areas of the country—that the news media has often missed. Instead, it has focused on how people who can still afford to buy groceries are switching to online and delivered venues, and the ways restaurants offer curbside pickup of meals and grocery packages.

As an ironic aside, Geoffrey Fowler, tech writer for the Washington Post, says that online ordering and curbside pickup saves a big chunk of the logistical cost of food buying for those who can afford it.[11] I say, why not just put in an order to yourself and pick up your fresh veggies "gardenside," saving an even bigger chunk of shopping logistical costs. That would also allow you to avoid "Amazon guilt," the feeling you get watching a gig worker risk their safety delivering your grocery package to a drop-off point while you wait safely inside your car or home.

Although Cotlon described his store as a happy place, and himself as optimistic, he said life in his neighborhood is hard jobs, long hours, bad pay, no health insurance, no money, poor diet, disabilities, and sickness. Meanwhile, his customers tend to buy snacks, candy, cold drinks, nachos with cheese, and cigarettes, because fruits and veggies are expensive.

That's what is so heartbreaking—because there really is an alternative to areas with limited access to affordable and nutritious food, especially those in predominantly lower-income communities. What these areas could really use is a lot more of the kind of backyard gardens I saw in my grandmother's neighborhood, as well as individual or shared plots in community gardens.

There is a Ninth Ward Community Garden, but it's in the Upper Ninth Ward, across the Industrial Canal and some thirteen blocks from the closest edge of the Ward. No Lower Ninth Ward community garden is registered with the American Community Gardening Association, which lists some four thousand community gardens across the U.S., but only fifteen in New Orleans. At one time the city had 154 such gardens,[12] most likely before hurricane Katrina in 2005 and about six other hurricanes since then. It's hard to grow gardens in a city hit by repeated hurricanes, you say? Of course, but I'd be willing to bet that in most cases, in most areas, it would provide a much more reliable food source than what Cotlon's customers have access to now.

Community gardens are usually organized into separate plots tended either by individuals for their own harvest or shared with others, or by those who want to donate their produce to food pantries. But they're often more than that, providing places where people come together to grow food, learn new skills, meet new people, and be an active part of their community. Since it's an outdoor activity, it's safer during the pandemic than indoor gatherings, or buying food in grocery stores for that matter.

Fact is, community and home gardens complement one another. In some ways community gardens are even better, as picking green beans and chatting side by side with a friend (that is, as side-by-side as you can get with masks and social distancing) offers just the kind of inspiration some people need to become active growers. By contrast, others treasure time alone in their gardens, communing in solace with the plants, bees, and soil. Different strokes for different folks.

Community gardens provide more than reduced costs, better taste, and increased consumption of freshly-grown vegetables and fruits. They also improve social health and cohesion, reduce stress, elevate mood, and enhance physical and mental health. And there's more. Studies show that they increase social activity for seniors, teach basic vocational skills, empower youth, and reduce crime and drug activity. They also create income activities, encourage water conservation and waste reduction, beautify the neighborhood, and even increase site and property values.[13]

Whether it's in a community garden or your back yard, if you're just starting for the first time, gardening does require inspiring yourself to learn how to do it. If you don't have a sunny yard and there's no community garden nearby, you may need to organize a neighborhood effort, find a vacant lot, and raise a little money—with a small grant, crowd-funding, bake sales, whatever. *The Community Gardening Handbook*, by Ben Raskin (Ilumina, 2017) and the American Community Gardening Association provide ideas and guidelines for getting started. In other words, you don't necessarily have to wait for good things to happen; make them happen yourself.

Already, there have been other encouraging responses to the decreased availability of food. Community supported agriculture enterprises (CSAs) are seeing a notable uptick in some places around the country. Surprisingly, these kinds of operations actually decreased following the 2008 recession, and evidently didn't recover. But new ones seem to be springing up. Organic sales have also increased, along with conventional grocery sales, though neither of those help the low-income very much. Other local venues, such as food hubs, urban farms, shared plots in community gardens, and farmers markets, will likely also register an increase in interest as the pandemic rages on.

I see all these alternatives to conventional food as highly desirable, but home food gardens should be the solid, most reliable anchor of a new food system. Just because they allow people to raise as much their own food as they can, rather than depending on other sources—even local—that may or may not be available in the coming months or years, for whatever reason.

Re-establish control over our food

You may not have thought of disempowerment as having anything to do with food. Well, it does, in several ways. The first is feeling powerless to overcome food insecurity, whether it's due to being chronically poor or suddenly being laid off with bleak prospects ahead. But when it comes to disempowerment, food insecurity addressed by handouts from food banks, noble as they are for helping hungry people, is only a temporary solution. It doesn't address the hunger for dignity and self-sufficiency as well as for food.

This is where food sovereignty comes in: that is, taking healthy ownership of, identification with, and power over where your food comes from and how it's produced. It puts those who grow and consume food at the heart of the food system rather than corporate profits, wherein a small handful of corporations control most of our food production, processing, and distribution. Food sovereignty is typically framed in terms of local food systems that usually don't include home gardens.

Yet, freedom from depending on others to produce and provide your food is the ultimate expression of food sovereignty and the answer to food insecurity. Or, in the case of food pantries, freedom from depending indefinitely on others' generosity when you're hungry. It's much better to grant yourself control of being generous to yourself, so to speak. And that means growing as much of your own food as you reasonably can, whether it's in your yard or on your patio or in a plot of your own in a community garden.

Wouldn't it be better to have a system in which home gardens play a major role, backed up by local producers and complemented by more distant or large-scale vendors, to supply items that can't easily be produced at home or locally? Of these three tiers, home gardens should be considered the most important simply because they're the least susceptible to catastrophic disruption. They could be the powerful backbone that anchors the entire system, especially during a crisis. In the words of Steve Solomon, "For people going through hard times, a thriving veggie garden can be the difference between painful poverty and a much more pleasant existence."

The second type of disempowerment goes deeper: it's having no idea whatsoever what it means to be truly and fully food-empowered, which affects all income levels, from pennyaires to billionaires. It's about a fundamental lack of genuine connection to your food.

Most people tend to think that as long as they're eating healthy food (if they are, which is often not the case), it doesn't matter who's growing it, where it's grown, or who prepares it. This is a misconception, a culturally-ingrained form of disempowerment resulting from our techno-mechanical way of life that's been foisted on us from the time we're toddlers. We're unaware that we've been ... separation-indoctrinated, for lack of a better term. That is, we've been separated from our essential human nature in many ways, not just in the nature of our relationship to food. And that matters, even if we've lost sight of it.

To better understand why, it helps to know how your physical body is constructed on a daily basis, which brings up another most-people-think fallacy. They think, Oh sure, my body comes from the plants and (if they're not vegetarian) plant-consuming animals that I eat. Okay, so far so good. But where do the plants come from? Most people would say, "Well, the ground, of course."

Wrong. Or technically, 99% wrong. The reason is that plants take in carbon dioxide, water, and sunshine to make sugar, giving off the oxygen in the process. This is photosynthesis, the chemical reaction that drives all life. And it's that sugar (converted into cellulose and other plant content), that's the source of 99% of the dry weight of a plant; less than 1% consists of minerals derived from the soil. To make it graphic, a block of dry wood is by weight 99% a block of an invisible gas—carbon dioxide—that's been mostly converted into solids, cellulose and lignin.

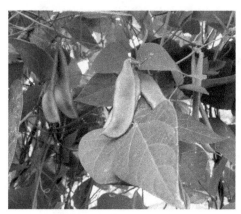
Photosynthesis in action

So a plant, any plant, comes 99% from air and sunshine. Especially when you consider that water taken up from the soil also comes from the air in the form of rain or snow. As I used to tell my students, "Do you like to eat? Do you like to breathe? Then you should thank photosynthesis every day."

Now, when you eat, you concentrate some of those soil-derived minerals, so that "only" 94% of your body weight comes from the air. Even then, the water you take in, which constitutes 62% of your weight, still comes indirectly from air-derived precipitation. Almost all of the rest is from the carbon dioxide, water, and nitrogen that comes from the air. So, to put it poetically (but accurately), your fabulous body is transformed vapor and sunlight, with a smidgen of flavoring from the soil. And all of the energy that you use to do anything—to kiss, to climb a mountain, to read a book, to think—is just transformed sunlight.

Growing your own food, then cooking and eating it, continues the marvelous transformation of photosynthesis. It's an act of creation and self-empowerment like no other. Absolutely no one should miss out on it. It should be taught over and over, with active participation in school gardens, from kindergarten through college. Yes, it's fine to mostly let others grow and prepare your food if you want. But if you never get the deep satisfaction of nurturing the whole process yourself, from earth-, air-, and sunshine-enabled seed all the way through to your taste buds, you will be missing a magical element of what it means to be human. As home gardener Sonnet Fitzgerald described it on Quora:

"There is something so amazing about starting to cook dinner, realizing you don't have anything in the freezer you want to make, and then just walking out the back door and gathering up a handful of carrots or peas or beans or spinach or salad. Just *right there*. Alive and warm and growing and smelling like sunshine. Then you rinse it in cold clean water and prep it and eat it like 15 minutes later. It's a feeling like nothing else."

Of course, this assumes that you garden in a way that isn't forced, tokenized, debilitating, or guilt-driven. And most importantly, that you enjoy. Because it has to feel personally fulfilling to experience the humanizing magic. That is, it needs to be *energizing*. It's something to consciously, gracefully allow, and not allowing it is a form of self-disempowerment, even if it's unintentional.

The third kind of disempowerment is about the exploitation of farm workers, meatpackers, and other workers the food system depends on. These people have been intentionally and systematically disenfranchised, dating back to antebellum times.

Itinerate farm workers in the U.S., the great majority of whom are immigrants, are struggling because of low pay, job uncertainty, unhealthy working conditions, low or no health insurance, and few if any benefits. They have high rates of respiratory disease, few legal options, and a real fear of speaking up. Yet they have to continue working hard during the COVID-19 pandemic as newly-designated "heroes," because without them we wouldn't be eating industrial food.

Industrial farm owners and meat- and poultry-packing companies claim that they're improving working conditions. But their response so far has been to rush into place minimal and often cosmetic changes needed to continue production, even at reduced capacity. They also keep workers in the dark as to how many of their comrades have been hit by, or even died from, the virus.

More than 24,000 COVID-19 cases had been tied to meatpacking plants as of June 16, 2020.[14] By Sept 13, at least 42,534 meatpacking workers had tested positive for COVID-19 in 494 meat plants, and at least 203 meatpacking workers had died since March, while regulators did almost nothing.[15] Even though some plants began operating again with plastic or steel partitions installed between work stations, temperature checks at the door, scattered break times, and paid leave for sick employees, these precautions haven't helped as much as the industry would like us to believe. One of the reasons is that Hispanic populations (the source of most workers) live in close quarters and are often packed into buses for transportation, the close proximity continuing to generate contagion at a high rate.

Meat- and poultry-packing companies have little intention of raising the working and living standards of their employees to that of the average American worker. They fear a significant increase in the cost of their products, which indeed has happened. That's why they're looking at the aforementioned increased robotics, AI (artificial intelligence), block chain technology, and automation to help replace virus-prone workers.

According to Ricardo Salvador of the Food and Environmental Program at the Union of Concerned Scientists, this whole system is modeled on antebellum plantation economics, just a step up from slavery. Or not—a step up, that is. Says a line worker at a notorious Mountaire plant in the hyper-hazardous poultry processing industry that pays 44% less than the national average for manufacturing jobs, "It's slavery, baby."[16]

Contrary to what you might hope for, the agriculture industry is exploiting the stress and confusion of the pandemic to reduce wages that are already so low, with working conditions so hazardous, that few Americans will take ag-worker jobs. As a result, this kind of employment continues to be left mostly to vulnerable immigrants so desperate for work they'll tolerate almost anything. The current industry language, says Salvador, is to refer to these workers as "inputs" like machinery, fertilizer, and pesticides, rather than employees who deserve a safe, healthy, and dignified livelihood. The Secretary of Agriculture (as of 2020) even framed pandemic-triggered worker pay cuts as "wage relief for farmers" in order to reduce costs. And the affected workers have virtually no bargaining power, having been forced to sign paperwork that says they are there only to do the work, then go home.

The Occupational Health and Safety Administration (OSHA) has been of virtually no help during the pandemic, even though its federal mandate is to protect employees from "recognized hazards." By July 7, 2020, it had issued only one citation resulting from more than six thousand COVID-19-related workplace complaints. This indicates that under the 2020 Administration the Labor Department would side with employers if workers sued.[17] Such is the face of farm, meat, poultry, and other food worker disempowerment.

In a home-garden anchored system, I predict that abused agricultural workers would gradually shift from the industrial to the local food system. There, they would likely be more valued and treated more humanely. The conglomeration of CSAs, urban farms, small local and community farms, food hubs, and—overlapping with home gardens—community gardens, is already in place and expanding. Others workers, with their considerable farming expertise, may want to start up their own local farms. A good example is Jorge's Market, the Latino family business just north of Fairfield, Iowa, which started up its own CSA after years of family members working on farms.[18] Perhaps some workers would become valued teachers for home gardeners or in schools. It could happen if we got out of the mindset that the industrial food system alone, or even local food systems, have to do everything.

Provide us with better nutrition

Unknown to most food shoppers, supermarket vegetables and fruits (as well as meats) have lost sizable amounts of nutrition over the last 70 years of conventional agriculture. Also at fault is the industrial degradation of soils, which have lost about half of their topsoil due to erosion, and of what's left, half of the organic matter that's essential to healthy plant growth. Altogether, that leaves only about a fourth of the original organic matter that remains. Thus, decades of degradation have brought about lower mineral levels in the soil, which tranform into reduced nutrient levels in the produce. And that, in turn, translates into less nutrients for customers, as noted in Chapter 2. Not only that, lower nutrient levels mean a blander taste. No wonder the number one reason most gardeners give for growing their own food is to improve taste.

Nutrition losses have been startling. A study of 43 vegetables and fruits published in 2004 revealed that between 1950 and 1999 reliable declines had occurred in the amounts of protein, calcium, phosphorus, iron, riboflavin (vitamin B2) and vitamin C.[19] A follow-up analysis of nutrient data from 1975 to 1997 found that calcium levels had dropped 27%, iron 37%, vitamin A 21%, and vitamin C 30% in twelve vegetables.[20] Another found that between 1930 and 1980, calcium had declined 19% and iron 22% in 20 vegetables.[21] And yet another reported that you would have to eat eight oranges today to get the same amount of Vitamin A as your grandparents would have gotten from one.[22]

The average distance between where food is grown and where it's eaten—1,500 miles—adds to these losses. The longer the time between harvest and consumption, the greater the nutrient loss. For instance, post-harvest loss of Vitamin C ranges from 15% in green peas to 77% for green beans. Spinach, by the time it's bought in a grocery store, has lost 90% of its Vitamin C and 50% of its folate and carotenoids.[23]

A fourth source of nutrient loss has been the replacement of healthy food with ultra-processed foods high in calories, salt, fat, and sugar but low in essential minerals, vitamins, and phytonutrients such as antioxidants. As mentioned earlier, fresh produce is sometimes not available at all, or is too expensive for many in low-income urban areas. The loss of market share in sit-down restaurants that has gone to fast-food chains since the pandemic broke out doesn't help.

Everyone agrees that nutrition is important, but few realize just how deficient we are in that regard. CNN, in a report entitled *The U.S. Food System is Killing People*, noted "the exceedingly poor baseline health of our country's population." Among our diet-related risk factors are chronic diseases such as hypertension, heart disease, and excessive calorie intake. About 70% of us now are overweight, including 40% who are obese. As mentioned previously—and it does bear repeating—about half of U.S. adults have diabetes or pre-diabetes, and only 12% of us are metabolically healthy with optimal levels of blood markers and pressures as well as a healthy body mass index.

Part of the history of this sad state of affairs began in the 1940s, when the government discovered that 40% of the country's young men were not physically fit to serve in the wartime military due to being malnourished and underweight. The resulting postwar industrialization of agriculture led to a food system that came to emphasize the highly processed, fat and carbohydrate-laden convenience foods and restaurant fare that we see today. Calorie-rich but nutrient-poor food is everywhere, with obesity beginning as early as age two. So we went from being underweight and malnourished to overweight and malnourished. The astonishing result: today 71% of 17 to

24 year-old men are unfit for military duty. Alarming as it was, we were better off being skinny.

Most, if not all, of this nutrition loss could be restored by emphasizing fruits and vegetables that have not been bred mostly for long-distance shipping and handling, are raised in healthy instead of degraded soil, grown as close as a few feet and minutes away from your table instead of thousands of miles away, and not processed into calorie-dense, nutrition-sparse fast food. In other words, food grown fresh in your own back yard, or at most within a few miles of your home.

Circumvent questionable food safety

Industrial Food often claims that U.S. food is "the safest in the world," yet the Centers for Disease Control and Prevention estimate that one in six people in the U.S. get food-borne illness every year, with 128,000 individuals hospitalized and 3,000 dying.[24]

The main areas of concern are pathogens, synthetic chemicals, pesticides, preservatives, antibiotics, and GMOs, with children being particularly vulnerable. The following is just the tip of the iceberg as to what could be said about shortfalls in food safety.

Pathogens

Between 2013 and 2018, the number of U.S. food recalls increased by 10%. Class I recalls—based on a "reasonable probability" that contaminated food could cause health problems—of meat and poultry rose by 8% during that time period.[25]

That pace has continued. "Much like 2018, last year [2019] seemed to experience a heightened number of food recalls—so much so that there seems to be some level of fatigue."[26] Those recalls were due to undeclared allergens, *Listeria, Salmonella, and E. Coli*, and foreign materials, mostly plastic and metal, some of which were present in Romaine lettuce as well as meats.[27] One reason for the increase of meat contamination may be that some industrial plants now allow the USDA to inspect up to 175 chickens per minute, up from 140 per minute recently.

Says Jaydee Hanson, of the Center for Food Safety,

"Officially, it's all still being inspected. But it's being inspected at such a high rate of speed that you can't really say it's being inspected . . . I have no idea how they could possibly inspect 170-some chickens going by a minute. The chicken's got to be bright orange or something to get pulled off the line."[28]

In case you're not mentally doing the math, that's about a third of a second for someone to inspect every conventionally raised piece of chicken you eat. Yet the USDA assures us that it has a "zero tolerance policy for fecal matter on meat and poultry." Fecal matter (i.e., poop) is where most bacterial contamination comes from. The problem is, official detection by the inspector applies only to fecal matter that's "visible" on the production line. At a third of a second per bird. Right.

Synthetic chemicals

Hundreds of chemicals have been added to processed foods, a source of contention for decades. But kids are especially vulnerable. The American Academy of Pediatrics has identified five chemical groups of concern for children: bisphenols (like BPA) that line metal cans; phthalates; perfluoroalkyl chemicals, perchlorate (found in food packaging); and nitrates/nitrites (curing agents present in some meats). These chemicals and others in our food (e.g., methylmercury and heavy metals) have been linked to developmental and reproductive harms, thyroid disruption, and cancer, but they're allowed in foods without any evidence base to show they're safe for youngsters, especially toddlers.[29] Not to mention what these chemicals might be doing to us adults, who are not exactly off the hook.

Pesticides

There are currently more than 68 pesticides used on food crops in the U.S., with seven of them classified as known carcinogens, and the rest as probable or possible carcinogens. As with non-pesticide chemicals used in food production, children are the most at risk. They are not simply "little adults," since their organs, nervous systems, and immune systems are still developing, making them especially vulnerable to toxic compounds. Unfortunately, most toxicity research is based on estimates of adult tolerance, simply because no one wants to use children as guinea pigs. Yet by allowing known and possible carcinogens into the food stream without adequate testing to account for the higher sensitivity of kids, that's exactly what we're doing to our children.

The most widely used pesticide, glyphosate, was designated in 2015 as a "probable" cause of cancer by the World Health Organization. Although its maker, Monsanto (now merged with Bayer), has long denied its carcinogenicity, the company recently agreed to pay more than $10 billion to tens of thousands of claimants that glyphosate caused non-Hodgkin's lymphoma. FDA chemist Richard Thompson wrote in a released email that most common U.S. foods had "a fair amount" of glyphosate in them.

Of course, glyphosate is just one of many pesticides that have been used in U.S. industrial agriculture for decades. Even with a number of those now banned, we still use 85 pesticides so toxic they've been banned or are in the process of being phased out in the European Union, China, or Brazil. Our top 12 fruits and vegetables with the most pesticide residues are, in order: strawberries, spinach, kale, nectarines, apples, peaches, cherries, pears, tomatoes, celery, and potatoes.

Organic, anyone? That would help, as organic fruits and vegetables average much lower levels of pesticides than conventional. Yet even some organic-certified produce has residues due to pesticide drift from conventional fields, processing errors in long food supply chains, or outright fraud.

Antibiotics

Today, almost all concentrated animal feeding operations (CAFOs) use antibiotics either in their food or water. Antibiotics are the modern "miracle" drugs that have helped fend off many bacterial diseases. Yet, rather than being used only to make up for unhealthy, crowded living conditions in CAFOs and to treat sick animals, they're mostly used as growth hormones, causing the animals to gain weight faster, and to attain a greater final weight, than they would otherwise. Antibiotics have been used on such a large scale that they've had a very unfortunate effect: by "leaking" into the food supply, they've contributed greatly to antibiotic resistance in humans. That means that over time, antibiotics have become less and less effective for sick people, so that when we really need them to treat a disease, resistant pathogenic bacteria readily overcome them. In 2016 the United Nations declared antibiotic resistance to be the most urgent global risk.[30]

U.S. producers are gradually beginning to reduce their use of agricultural antibiotics, but with so many loopholes and misleading practices that it often amounts to business as usual. For instance, McDonald's announced that they would use only chickens that were raised "without antibiotics that are important to human medicine." However, the self-prohibited human drugs they're talking about are not currently approved for use in food animals anyway. Moreover, the new policy does nothing to reduce antibiotics important to human medicine that are used on other livestock.[31] Meanwhile, the E.U. uses far fewer antibiotics than the U.S., and has banned many U.S. meat products because we still use them.

In any case, growing your own fruits and vegetables eliminates 99% of food safety problems. As for animal protein, unless you want to keep a few hens for eggs or go the Kingsolver route and raise some poultry for meat, you might still have to rely on local farms for fresh animal protein. Mostly likely because of their small size, local organic farms evidently have far fewer problems with food safety than CAFOs and other industrial farms.

GMOs

Absolutely nothing in the entire food arena is more contentious than genetically modified organisms (which now includes "gene-edited" crops). It's as controversial as the abortion debate. Despite the fact that numerous articles and books have thoroughly documented the industry and scientific fraud that vaulted genetically engineered corn, soybeans, canola, sugar beets, and cotton into widespread use, it is still fiercely defended by many (but far from all) academics and the agro-industrial complex. The use of GMOs pits two antithetically opposite worldviews against one another: one that values genuinely natural processes above all, and the other that believes that anything goes regardless of how unnatural it is, with each claiming that sound science is on its side. Scientists with relevant expertise who object to the way the GMO venture has been conducted on scientific and regulatory grounds have been accurately conveying the facts and upholding the other standards of science. By contrast, scientists promoting GMOs have significantly misrepresented key facts and dishonored other scientific standards. Due to billions of dollars in industry advertising and lobbying, the pro-GMO side has prevailed in terms of adoption, even though a majority of the public has safety concerns and believe GMOs should at least be clearly labeled. That desire has been repeatedly thwarted by the industrial food industry, which has resulted in private non-GMO certification efforts.

Nevertheless, no comprehensive, scientifically-controlled safety testing of human subjects has ever been done on the major GMO food crops, for the inescapable reason that any such attempt by a university researcher would spell the end of their career. That is, assuming the National Science Foundation or the USDA would approve funding for such research, which is highly unlikely. For controlled human testing, which could have been done decades ago, it's a story of continued academic "don't ask don't tell." That, of course, is not responsible science at all. Such is the fierceness of the prevailing academic and political dogma that GMOs are safe. The situation is an exact replay of the decades in which a wide range of toxic pesticides and other chemicals were claimed by the agro-chemical industry to be "scientifically" proven as safe, only to see them banned once the evidence of harmful health and environmental effects became too obvious to further deny.

But the tide may be turning, as the blockbuster glyphosate case against Monsanto/Bayer has indicated. Glyphosate use had exploded after corn and soybeans were genetically engineered to tolerate it so that it could be used to control weeds without ostensibly harming the crop. Already questioned for some time by scientists and regulators in Europe, where it is largely banned, its long-repeated claims of health and environmental safety are now being steadily discredited in this country as well. Part of the reason is that GMO crops are increasingly subject to massive insect and weed resistance, rendering them less and less useful and more costly as farmers turn to regenerative strategies. All of which has led to predictions of the coming obsolescence of GMO seeds.[32]

Overall, the reason GMOs and the other categories of industrial safety lapses have persisted is that Big Food tends to favor sales over safety. Typically, they use "the playbook," a set of tactics borrowed from the tobacco and the climate-change denying oil industry. Longtime nutrition expert Marion Nestle says that when dealing with signs that our food isn't as safe or nutritious as it claims, the industry's plan is to cast doubt on unhelpful science; fund more favorable, skewed science; offer gifts and consultancies to food researchers; sponsor professional bodies; and use front groups posing as independent institutes. Also, to promote personal responsibility and self-regulation rather than government intervention; capture advisory committees; and challenge regulation in court.[33]

Of course, none of the above includes perhaps the worst safety threat of all: the obesity epidemic. How can the industrial food system claim to deliver safe food when it has produced a population of which 70% is overweight or obese, with nearly 50% diabetic or pre-diabetic? With all the misery and expense it takes to deal with those and other chronic, diet-related threats?

So, safest food in the world? Or to use the industry's clever hedge, among the safest in the world? That is, compared to other countries that employ the same, highly-compromised industrial food system?

Need we lay out in detail how home gardens vastly improve on all those safety concerns? It's pretty simple: no pathogens, synthetic chemicals, pesticides, risky preservatives, antibiotics, or GMOs.

Make food readily accessible without abusing food workers

Food production has been a story of not just continued but intensified food worker exploitation since the onset of COVID-19. Why should these people now be proclaimed as "essential" and "heroes," even though they're evidently still not necessary and heroic enough to be accorded safe working conditions with decent pay and benefits?

A significant expansion of home food gardens would present the industry with a stark choice: either address the plight of food workers like you mean it, or they will seek better working conditions in home and local food arenas when the great food shift starts gathering a real head of steam. Meanwhile, growing and harvesting vegetables from home and community gardens will not endanger the food workers—that is, gardeners—who grow them.

Retain maximum flexibility in challenging times

The pandemic has revealed an industrial system that has found it difficult to divert food from restaurants, schools, and hotels to grocery stores and food pantries. As noted earlier, farmers have been forced to plow under or otherwise dispose of good food, and to euthanize millions of pigs, chickens, and cattle; they now struggle to re-imagine their operations. Moreover, cars line up for miles as people wait their turn at the food pantries because they can't afford the food in grocery stores. And only a small percentage of those who need food can get it from pantries, which lack sufficient storage and distribution capacity to reach all those who have little other choice.

Food shoplifting has spiked during the pandemic.[34] Typical of such shoplifters is a woman who lost her receptionist job but didn't qualify for unemployment. She then gave up on local food banks because of the long lines. Desperate, she resorted to sneaking ground beef, rice, and potatoes into her son's stroller, telling herself that God would understand. And She might.

By contrast, a fully unleashed home garden-anchored system is the most flexible means of food production, as it's the only one in which have people have immediate control over their food. Maximum flexibility also means greatly increased backup in a pinch. Even if you lose your job, a healthy garden keeps on growing. Or if it's winter and you're well stocked up from your summer garden, you can continue to draw on that bounty until you replant. Even a winter garden (see Chapter 8) can help out. Plus, a neighborhood full of thriving gardens fosters learning among neighbors, swapping harvested foods, and mutual support when things go wrong. Instead of when the going gets tough, the tough go shopping, it's when the going gets tough, the tough start planting.

Cause no environmental damage

As you will recall, the industrial food system totes up to at least $3 trillion in global environmental damage, of which at least $16 billion is incurred by U.S. domestic and imported vegetable production. Meanwhile, most home gardens incur zero such damage. Just think of what we could do if even 1% of those billions was diverted into fostering home and community gardens.

Transform food production from a huge net carbon emitter to a net carbon sink

When you include all causes, from soil loss and degradation to food waste, and to the transport, refrigeration, freezing, processing and packaging of food, about 43-57% of all greenhouse gas emissions are due to industrial food production.[35] All of which is rapidly warming the planet and causing climate change. I mentioned earlier that industrial farming has stripped away about half of our topsoil due to wind and water erosion and, to add insult to injury, robbed the remaining soil of about half of its organic matter.

Lost organic matter really matters, as it represents a vast reservoir of carbon. Growing plants in a way that regenerates soil, as home gardens do over time, also restores carbon in the form of organic matter. Rattan Lal, a soil scientist at Ohio State University, estimates that changes in soil management could coax up to two-thirds of all the carbon lost from soils back underground, significantly reducing atmospheric carbon dioxide.[36] This could help transform agricultural soil from being a net carbon emitter to a net sink, which would help cool down the planet.

Interestingly, sequestering soil carbon need not be limited to just restoring what's been lost. Some gardening and farming methods rapidly infuse so much compost into the soil (e.g., biodynamics) that it could quickly double the amount carbon that was in the soil prior to modern agriculture. This would be a far cheaper, safer, more soil-beneficial, and healthier method of recapturing carbon than high-tech capture-and-storage methods. According to a 2019 study in the journal *Science*, planting a trillion trees could sequester about 225 billion tons of carbon, or about two-thirds of the carbon released by humans into the atmosphere since the Industrial Revolution began.[37] That would be a good start. If farming and gardening removed another 10-20%, we'd be most of the way toward pre-industrial levels. Or maybe even better. Recent reports from farming systems and pasture trials around the world show that regenerative organic agriculture could sequester 100% of current CO2 emissions.[38]

So yes, growing your own little—or maybe not so little—garden helps to cool us off. When you consider the scores of millions of such gardens that already exist in the U.S. alone, and how much they could expand in both area and number, you can see how it could help not only yourself and your family and country, but also the whole planet.

Transition quickly, smoothly, and economically to a far healthier and more accessible supply of food

So to put it all together, home gardens are well-positioned to implement all of the proposed improvements to industrial food, and in a timely manner. It is so needed, not only during this pandemic but, as we're hearing more and more often, possible future pandemics. It's hard to imagine the industrial food system effectively addressing any one of these concerns, let alone most or all of them, much less as quickly and easily as a home-garden anchored system can. And, I predict, will.

4

Why Industrial Food Can't Match the Efficiency of Home Gardens

Let's face it: with few exceptions the media continue to push the narrative that the U.S. industrial food system is almost magically efficient. Yet by now you may be starting to see that when all the costs and benefits are included in the reckoning, it can't even begin to compete with the efficiency of a home garden-anchored system. But wait, as of 2019, the U.S. food system, including food service and food retailing, was truly gargantuan—over $6 trillion per year.[1] How could home gardens come anywhere near making a significant dent in that market?

Scope

First, let's consider the parameters of a meaningful comparison. For home gardens we're talking mainly about fruits and vegetables. That's only a small fraction of an agricultural market that includes animal-based products, grains, and soybeans, with much of the grains and soy going to animal feed, fuel tanks, and industrial uses other than food. For what's left, the most useful evidence that home gardens can have a big impact is—once again—supplied by the 40% of vegetables grown in the 20 million victory gardens in 1944. That was about one garden for every seven people. If there had been even just two gardens for every seven people, it would have had the potential to double the proportion of U.S. vegetable production to 80%. That would have allowed conventional agriculture to focus more on meat, dairy, and grains, which are not amenable to producing in back yards.

Could we do something like 80% or more now? No reason why not, assuming that the ratio between commercial and home production efficiency hasn't changed much since 1944. Forty percent of vegetable production today, at the rate of one garden for every seven people, would involve about 47 million gardens. According to the National Gardening Association, we already have about 43 million such gardens. And since about 100 million homes have lawns, and as they're about thirty times as large as the average 15' x 20' food garden, space is not a barrier to expansion. In fact, those lawns occupy about 40 million acres,[2] which works out to 5,260 square feet of potential garden area for every man, woman, and child in the U.S. And since collectively lawns are the largest irrigated crop in the country,[3] and as vegetables need a good amount of water, we'd be all set. That is, if that lawn area could somehow be distributed to everyone who wanted a garden, which of course is not possible in densely-populated cities. Still, it gives an indication of the huge potential of lawns.

If increased home food production could be quickly ramped up in the 1940s, it could be quickly increased again, covering possibly an even greater proportion of food needs. Remember, Nigeria, with far less in the way of developed resources than we have, produces 50% of its food in home gardens on only 2% of its cropland. Not to be outdone, Cuba produces 60% of all its vegetables in urban gardens. Similar numbers are enjoyed by other developing countries.[4] If people in those countries can do such things, why couldn't we?

The amount of food grown at home could range anywhere from a tomato plant in a patio container to the current 15' x 20' average garden to much more. As mentioned earlier, common estimates of the garden area needed to feed one person for a year range from 4,000 to 6,000 square feet. Or, to feed a family of four, about a fourth of an acre (10,890 sq. ft.), slightly larger than the average size of the American lawn. Maybe in some cases a third of an acre would be required. Other estimates say much less is needed. It really depends on a host of variables, including gardening experience, soil fertility, the plants grown, the methods used, climate, and available water.

The global average is 0.5 acre/person.[5] By contrast, it takes about three acres to feed one American (discussed in more detail in Chapter 8). Yet, of the 392 million acres of U.S. cropland, only 6.6 million acres are used to grow the commercially-produced vegetables we consume. Given our population of 331 million, industrial vegetable production thus requires just 0.02 acres/person (6.6 million acres/331 million people), which is 871 square feet, a plot measuring only 30' x 30'. Sounds impressive compared to the 6,000 square feet (77' x 77') some claim you need to grow your own, right?

Not really.

Category 1 and 2 foods

To explain why, I first need to designate vegetables, fruits, and legumes as Category 1 foods and how they, along with Category 2 foods (described below), would fit into a three-tiered system. Category 1 includes calorie- and nutrient-rich corn, winter squash, potatoes, sweet potatoes, and beans, as well as low-calorie but nutrient-rich veggies like leafy greens, tomatoes, peppers, and carrots. Other unprocessed or minimally-processed whole foods, such as locally-produced meat, fish, eggs, dairy, and grain products, could conceptually also be included. However, for the purposes of this discussion, I'll consider only fresh produce in Category 1. In any case, Category 2 is quite different. It consists of industrially-produced foods: ultra-refined grain products; fats and oils; meats, fish, eggs, and dairy; and sweeteners. According to the USDA, the average American diet, measured by calorie content, consists of 15% Category 1 and 85% Category 2 foods. So that 851 square feet of land producing all the vegetables consumed by an average person per year accounts for only 15% of their calorie intake. Calorie-wise, it would sustain them for only 15% of a year, or a little less than two months. So as it turns out, a 30' x 30' patch of land (900 sq. ft.) is not that impressive after all. That is, compared to a 77' x77' home garden (6,000 sq. ft.), the area some claim is needed to sustain a person for a whole year. We'll return to these figures shortly. And by the way, this is just a production comparison; I'm not suggesting that everyone needs to be a vegetarian.

I have not been able to find average U.S. calorie intakes for category 1 and 2 foods in USDA dietary data for 1945, but who knows, it may be buried somewhere in their archives. The fact that 40% of young men at that time were unfit for military service due to mal- and under-nourishment doesn't help much, as it indicates that they weren't getting enough of either category of food.

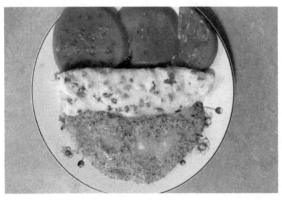

Category 1 (grits and tomatoes) and Category 2 (omelet) foods

What it all means is that for home gardens to comprise a meaningful source of healthy calories as well as non-calorie nutrients, we would need to do two things. First, greatly increase our consumption of Category 1 foods while decreasing the share of Category 2. Second, favor calorie- and nutrient-rich vegetables over nutrient-rich but calorie-sparse vegetables by a ratio of 2 to 1—just as recommended by the 1944 USDA Victory Garden Guide. Yet as mentioned previously, virtually all Category 1 foods grown in gardens today are of the low-calorie type. Which, nevertheless, could be a good dietary choice for those trying to lighten up, at least until they reached a healthier weight.

Fortunately, an increase in home gardens would require an increase in exercise and exposure to fresh air and nature. So a massive shift to a home-garden diet would result in a welcome move toward better health, conferring an added benefit that industrial food systems can't match. However, if we continue business as usual, with 85% of our calories coming mostly from ultra-processed grains, fats and oils, animal products, and sweeteners, we'd continue to contribute to the enormous external costs of industrial food production, as will be described shortly.

Those, among other factors described below, are what makes the home garden alternative so attractive. To again cite that highest estimate, a well-planned and tended 6,000 square feet vegetable garden could fulfill 100% of your nutritional needs with Category 1 foods for a year. That is, except for Vitamin

B12, unless you include some egg-laying hens in your garden. Even that relatively large amount of space provides nutrition far more efficiently than the three acres (130,680 sq. ft.) the industrial food system needs to feed you a combination of 15% Category 1 and 85% Category 2 foods.

On the other hand, you could decide to live on only fruits and vegetables, but with the industrial system as your supplier. At an average rate of 851 square feet of land required to supply 15% of your calories, it would take 5,673 square feet to provide 100% of your calories with the same kinds of Category 1 foods as are currently consumed. Notice how close that is to the 6,000 square feet some consider necessary to be food self-sufficient. As you will see in Chapter 5, it can require less than a fourth of that area, depending on yield and consumption rates and the amounts of Category 1 and Category 2 crops grown.

Not that we have to choose between all Category 1 food and the usual Category 1- and 2-combo. Maybe you (like me) aren't willing to go the vegetarian route, or to give up breads and pastries. Or to forego meats and dairy, although for many, eggs from a couple backyard hens are well within reach. Fine, you can rely on local farms and processors for grains and animal products. After all, some 8% of all farms are already producing local foods. So, even though they produce only a tiny percentage of all consumed food (much less than 8%), they're more available than you might think. And surely you (again, like me) don't want to give up bananas, pepper, chocolate, oranges, coffee, avocados, butter, olive oil, cinnamon, and other shipped-in goodies that make up maybe 5-10% of your diet. So for those kinds of items you'd continue to rely on a distantly-produced tier of the food system, ideally favoring organic, regenerative, and fair trade principles whenever you can.

External Costs

Even with a few nice "extras" from the industrial tier you'd still greatly decrease the real cost of feeding yourself mainly with a home garden. At the scale of the whole country, most of the savings would come from avoiding the enormous external costs incurred by the industrial food system.

External costs are not reflected in the price you pay at the checkout counter when you shop at a supermarket or convenience store, or pick up your curbside takeout at a restaurant. That's why they're called external. These costs to human health and safety are staggering: pesticide toxicity, water pollution, junk food that feeds the obesity epidemic, antibiotic resistance, and damage to the rural environment from soil depletion, erosion, and lost biodiversity. Loss of mid-sized farms and pollution of neighboring and downstream communities that contribute to negative social and economic impacts.

The multinational Food and Land Use Coalition estimates those costs globally at $12 trillion a year.[6] TruCost, a global risk-assessment service, reported in a study prepared for the UN that external environmental costs alone add up to $3 trillion annually[7]. Topping that, a 2004 study at Iowa State University arrived at a partial price tag of at least $4.97 trillion per year for the external costs of U.S. industrial agriculture[8]. An updated, full-cost accounting would surely reveal a considerably higher figure. Not to mention the $2.6 trillion annual cost to the U.S. economy caused by wasted food[9]. As an indication of how it would play out for business, KPMG, the giant multinational professional services network, determined that if external prices were internalized, they would equal at least 224% of the industry's revenue.[10] In other words, the costs they incur but don't pay are two and a quarter times their income.

External costs are picked up by taxes that pay for subsidies and public damages, higher insurance premiums to cover health costs of the diet-related chronic diseases mentioned earlier, and in many other ways.

To cite just one example, consider the massive amount of wasted fertilizer that runs off farm fields and into rivers, especially in the agriculture-intensive Midwest. In Iowa, the Des Moines Waterworks' nitrate-removal plant, the largest in the world, removes toxic nitrogen fertilizer from the city's drinking water, which comes in part from the Des Moines River. The plant was covered by the taxpayers who built it in 1992 at a cost of $9.2 million, upgraded its capacity at a price tag of $15 million in 2016, and now must maintain it at a total cost of some $1.5 million annually. The half-a-million people of the greater Des Moines area have no choice if they want safe water in their homes.

Excess fertilizer runoff from the Midwest also results in a 7,800 sq. mi. (the size of Massachusetts) "dead zone" in the Gulf of Mexico around the mouth of the Mississippi. It severely reduces water quality in that area every year. In that case, it's the fishing and tourism industries who pay external costs of $82 million a year in the form of lost income. In 2013, the Iowa Nutrient Reduction Strategy, at the direction of the Midwest Gulf Hypoxia Task Force, launched a "voluntary" program for farmers with the goal of reducing nitrogen and phosphorus runoff 45% by 2035. Yet in 2018 it reported that not only was nitrogen runoff not decreasing, it had increased by 34%.

As large as it is, fertilizer runoff represents just one tiny facet of the industrial food system's total cost outsourcing. Perhaps the most troubling is people eating way too much calorie-laden unhealthy food. We make a pretense at being concerned, putting most of the blame on overweight people for not getting enough exercise. Never mind industry efforts to make junk food as biologically addictive as cigarettes are physiologically compulsive, then suck people in with extraordinarily effective advertising. I haven't eaten junk food for quite a while, and I'm philosophically opposed to it. Yet when I'm watching an NBA game on TV and those fast-food commercials come on, they're so compelling I feel an almost overwhelming urge to jump up and rush out to get a juicy burger, tasty fries, and sugary soft drink. Even when I'm not hungry! I can imagine that fast food industry types reading this will chortle, congratulating themselves at how truly clever they are. Because if their ads can affect me that powerfully, the addiction-inducing effect on the average fast-food customer will be even greater. In fact, irresistible. Just what the industry wants and depends on for its business model.

The supposed antidote to all this outsourcing is true cost accounting, which has become somewhat of a cottage industry among those protesting external costs of industrial food production. However, the numerous studies that have explored it, while recognizing that the corporations behind it cannot make a profit if external costs were internalized and would thus never agree to significant change, still call for somehow restructuring it.[11] I say don't bother with trying to change a massive and deeply ossified system; it's a waste of time, a lost cause. Rather, simply plant the seeds of a new system by going all out to energize home and community gardens. The three-tiered, home garden anchored system has by far the greatest promise of efficiently moving us out of an otherwise hopeless situation.

Of course, we could just go on ignoring the fact that the real price of our food is far more than what we pay at the grocery store or restaurant. But why do that? To appropriate the Pointer Sisters' soulful lament in their 1974 hit *Fairytale*, it seems we've been lost in a dream. That is, we have deluded ourselves into believing the fairytale, the fantasy that industrial food is safe and cheap. It's time to wake up, with the COVID-19 pandemic shaking our shoulders and splashing a pitcher of cold water over our still-dreaming heads.

Wake up! Wake up! Wake up!

Energy Efficiency

Closely related to external costs is embodied energy, which is all the energy used in the creation of a product. In response to environmentalists' claims that local food systems are more energy-efficient, a number of studies have attempted to compare them to industrial food systems.[12] However, it is difficult to fully account for the energy embedded in the extraction, refinement, and use of fossil fuels, minerals and metals, as well as the manufacture and use of agricultural and processing machinery, road degradation by 18-wheelers, and the like. Not to mention the energy expended in dealing with all the health, environmental, economic, and social damage wrought by the trillions of dollars in external costs mentioned above. Yet even with limited consideration of energy requirements, for every calorie of food energy, industrial food uses 10 to 15 calories of production energy, which can be reduced by 90% when food is sourced within 12 miles of where it's produced.[13]

Local farms also require energy-consuming machinery, fuel, processing, and delivery that gardeners mostly don't need for home food production. Those costs—depending on the definition of local, which often extends to 400 miles from the point of consumption—likely reduce total energy consumption by a sizable factor even while equaling or improving food production per unit of land. Again, it's not that I'm in any way against local farms, CSAs, farmers markets, and the like. On the contrary, I'm all for them; they're the second tier of the system I propose.

Yes, growing it yourself does require the energy embedded in seed production, gardening supplies, fences, compost, a wheelbarrow, natural fertilizers, canning and freezing of perishables, etc. (However, it requires virtually no extra energy to store calorie-rich dried corn, beans, winter squash, and sweet- and Irish potatoes.) You could even count the embedded energy of your own labor. But it and all the other home energy costs are surely negligible, per unit of food produced, compared to the full, gargantuan total of that required by industrial food. Since money follows energy, see the cost comparison of home gardens versus industrial food in Chapter 3 to get an idea of the energy difference.

In any case—I can't emphasize it enough—if we exert ourselves wisely, it ends up being an energizing benefit rather than an energy cost in view of the often much-needed exercise, exposure to nature, and healthier food that we get when we grow a garden.

The three-tiered food system

Chapter 3 introduced the concept of home gardens as the anchor of a three-tiered system. Perhaps you can now more easily see—due to the enormous external costs of the industrial system—how such a system would out-perform the current, almost exclusively industrial model, hands down. That is, with home gardens providing mainly Category 1 foods, backed up by local and reduced industrial systems that supplement whatever people want in Category 1 or 2 foods but can't or prefer not to produce themselves. As mentioned above, meat, dairy, eggs, and grains that are un- or minimally processed would be available in the second tier of the system. The idea is that, in time, home gardens would supply much to most of our food needs, with local producers supplying somewhat less, and industrial or distant producers less still. The proportions of these tiers would be flexible depending on many factors, and would change over time. But a reliable constant would be that the national cost—external *and* internal—to operate the three-tiered system would be immensely lower than that of the current industrial system.

How much lower? Well, let's start with what we know. In 2019, about 33% of U.S. households raised food gardens, spending an estimated $3.76 billion.[14] At that rate, 100% of households would spend $11.3 billion. It takes about 4 sq. ft. per day to meet my nutritional needs (Table 5-5), which would require 1,460 sq. ft. per year. For the sake of argument, assume that the average person eats 50% more than I do; that would require 2,000 sq ft. (a plot of 44' x 44'), about a fifth of the average-sized lawn.

Since food gardens average 600 sq. ft. (25' x 25'), a plot measuring 2,000 sq. ft. would proportionately cost 3.3 times as much as gardeners currently spend, adding up to $37.7 billion per year. However, that figure is based on just one person per household, and there are an average of 2.5 persons per household. So multiply that $37.7 billion by 2.5, and you get $94.3 billion.

For nutritional self-sufficiency, assume that gardeners would favor calorie-rich beans, corn, potatoes, etc. to low-calorie tomatoes, carrots, greens, and such by a ratio of 2:1. Then, throw in $25 billion to cover costs of starting up new community gardens to accommodate people who don't have their own garden space; the total would then be $119.3 billion per year. In as much as internal and external costs of industrial food add up at least $4 trillion per year, the cost of home gardens for the whole country would be about 3% that of industrial food production. This, despite the fact that I intentionally inflated some of the expenses, such as the average person consuming 50% more than I would, and $25 billion (a generous guess) for new and expanded existing community gardens.

The first tier of self-sufficient food production in a three-tiered, home garden anchored food system would thus be vastly more cost-efficient than the industrial food system delivering the current American diet. Of course, not everyone is going to fully jump into that first tier, even though a third of the country is already in it, and another third is on its way. But to the degree that people do take that path, the cost of food production would go down proportionately, to as little as 3% of what we now spend. That's a possibility worth pondering.

5

Walking the Garden Talk

All my talk about the power of home gardening doesn't mean much if I haven't "been there and done that" in a way that could feasibly be repeated in millions of home gardens. It's the stamp of credibility to show that what I'm advocating is possible, both for individual gardeners and for inspiring the creation of a new food production system nationwide. My previous experience with growing vegetables occurred when I was more or less where most gardeners are now: interested, having fun, enjoying the fresh produce, but with no real thought of it providing much or possibly even most of my sustenance. Much less being part of a food-system remake of the country as a whole. However, with the emergence of the pandemic, I felt like I had to up my game. So I grew stuff and took notes.

Writing this book, mostly over the summer and fall of 2020, it was just so satisfying and rewarding to leave my computer from time to time to go out and tend my own garden, now that it had a bigger purpose. I assumed I'd have an absolutely abundant harvest that I'd then be able to triumphantly tout to inspire people.

It didn't one hundred percent work out that way. Some of the fourteen tomato plants died early from yellowing and withering (nutrient deficiency?), although enough did well to produce my best harvest ever. One plant, way over in a corner and crowded on two sides by tall poles of lush green beans and colored butter beans, grew spectacularly well, producing maybe 15 pounds of large, blemish-free tomatoes. It was still bearing ripe fruit in mid-October, right here in Iowa. Just 30 feet away from the early flame-outs, so go figure. Meanwhile, squash vine borers devastated the Red Kuri squash, so I got only 38 pounds. Equally disappointing were the two 24-foot rows of all-purple potatoes, which gave me a measly 28 pounds. As you'll see in a bit, the yield for those two crops should have been much higher.

The two rows of green beans, planted in hills around separate poles amidst the squash, surprised me. They grew very lush foliage, but no flowers for weeks; I thought they were never going to blossom and produce beans. Then, suddenly they took off, eventually yielding more than I ever expected. I think I might have given them too much compost and organic nitrogen fertilizer, because the leaves, though healthy green, were at first highly convex, not flat like they're supposed to be. That's often a sign of too much nitrogen. I'd never grown these varieties of squash, potatoes, and green beans before, and it showed. That's gardening: you learn something new every year.

On the other hand, I'd never grown sweet potatoes before either, but they produced an average 5.5 pounds per hill, despite the voles that devoured parts of some of them. I should probably attribute my success there to Steve Solomon's advice to mix some sand into the heavy clay soil, plant the slips in raised hills, and only lightly fertilize them with compost.[1] I also grew a mix of collards and various kinds of kale, planted in between some of the tomato plants. They far exceeded my expectations as well.

Interestingly, I got 0.95 portions per square foot of butter beans in 2020 using one double row, with the rows planted one foot apart, and 0.83 portions per square feet in 2018 from two rows 4 feet apart. (You'll see below what I mean by portions.) The 2020 crop was also half as much work, since I provided only one vertical lattice for the vines to climb on, compared to two in 2018. Although the rows were 24 feet long in both years, they were not wholly comparable, as I harvested almost all of the 2018 beans dry, and most of the 2020 beans fresh, the majority of which I froze.

With these results in mind, I'll now revisit the Chapter 2 measures by which to evaluate the worth of produce, this time applied to my (24' x 31') garden in 2020. I kept meticulous records of every ounce of every vegetable I harvested, so the math was easy.

- Cash value

  Based on the USDA's average retail price per pound of each vegetable, multiplied by the average industry premium of 70 percent more for organic, I harvested $603 worth of produce. I could have grown my own heirloom tomato starter plants, but opted instead to buy them, costing me $35. I also bought $10 worth of sweet potato slips, so my cash "profit" was $558, right in line with the examples of garden profits mentioned in Chapter 2.

- Weight

  The garden yielded 456 pounds of fresh produce (Table 5-2), about half of which was tomatoes. (In fact, counting the original weight of tomatoes before they were rendered down into sauce and frozen, the total was 535 pounds.) Yet the watery tomatoes provided only a small fraction of the calorie output of the corn, beans, potatoes, winter squash, and sweet potatoes, which again is why weight alone is misleading.

- Yield

  I harvested 535 pounds from my 24' x 31' plot, which equals 535 pounds per 744 square feet, which is 0.7 pounds per square foot. At that rate, I could expect to produce 30,492 pounds of vegetables on a full acre, despite the poor potato and winter squash yield rates.

- Survival value

  If you'll recall, this is how long how your garden would keep you alive if you had to depend on it for all your food. I've come up with a simple accounting system, which I'm calling portion-based, to assess that measure of worth.

Portion-based garden evaluation

Follow along on Tables 5-1 and 5-2 to get an idea of how the portion-based system works. The steps to arrive at your own portion-based measurements are listed below. I think this way of measuring is more useful than the usual strategy of simply listing average weight or volume per veggie per length of row, since that can vary so extensively for different people and different gardens.

Although it's all simple math, for those who are easily bored by numbers, I've provided key summary points at the beginning of each table so you can skip over the table itself. For those who want to know more, follow the text along with the figures.

How to calculate your portion-based garden yield:

1. Determine the numbers of portions of different kinds of foods you typically eat every day for breakfast, lunch, and supper (and perhaps more if you include between-meal snacks). For me, on average, it's three portions each for those three meals.

Table 5-1. 2018 (beans) and 2019 (corn) plots

Two plots, totaling 22' x 22', grew enough beans
and corn to last 55 days if that were all I ate.

Crop	Total harvest, lb.	Weight per portion, oz.	Portions available	Days harvest would last at 9 portions per day	Plot size, sq. ft.
Colored butter beans, dry	10.2	1.5	108.8	12.1	132
Corn - grits - dumplings	24.0 12.0	1.5 1.5	256.0 128.0	28.4 14.2	352
Total	46.2		492.8	54.7	484

2. Decide how much of any food item constitutes a fulfilling, healthy portion for you. For instance, Table 5-1 shows that 1.5 ounces of dried butterbeans, when hydrated and cooked, constitutes one portion for me. For Red Kuri winter squash (Table 5-2), it's 7 ounces, as it contains a lot more water than dried beans. In general, the pre-prep weight of calorie-dense veggies will be less than that of the calorie-sparse ones. But you can't just assume what will work; you'll have to determine the correct weights per portion by trying them out for yourself.

3. Divide the total weight of your harvested vegetable (or a garden average from the Internet if you haven't grown it yet) by the weight per portion to see how many portions the total harvest would provide, and thus how many days it would last you. For instance, my 2018 harvest of 10.2 pounds of dry butterbeans would yield 109 1.5-ounce portions. At nine portions per day, that would last about 12 days if I ate nothing but butterbeans three times a day (Table 5-1). Of course, I would never do that. The point is to provide a way to see how long my harvest would last when applied to all the crops I want to grow and eat.

For example, for lunch I might have one portion each of sweet potatoes, butterbeans, and greens. That would be two calorie-rich to one calorie-sparse food (both nutritious, by the way). You could mix and match any of the foods, any way you like, to provide your idea of an interesting, satisfying, and nutritious meal.

4. You can then use this system to see how large your garden would have to be in order to feed yourself for a year, given the amounts of each crop you grow and how well they yield. As you can see from Table 5-1, the corn and butterbeans I grew on a total of 484 square feet in 2018 and 2019 would last me about 55 days if that were all I ate. My 2020 garden (Table 5-2), grown on 744 square feet, would last me about 128 days. If I had grown it all in the same year, I would have had 183 days' worth of food (Table 5-3)—exactly half a year. After that, I'd have to head to the grocery store.

Table 5-2. 2020 Garden

A 21' x 34' plot grew enough vegetables to last me 128 days.

Crop	Total harvest, lb.	Weight per portion oz.	Portions available	Days harvest would last at 9 portions per day	Plot size sq. ft.
Potatoes	28.2	13.0	34.7	3.9	
Winter squash	35.7	7.0	81.6	9.1	
Sweet potatoes	66.5	8.0	133.0	14.8	
Butterbeans:					
frozen	13.0	3.2	65.0	7.2	
dry	1.4	1.5	14.9	1.7	
Green beans:					
canned	19.9	3.6	88.4	9.8	
frozen	9.1	3.6	40.4	4.5	
dry	1.3	1.5	13.9	1.5	
fresh	5.2	5.2	16.0	1.8	744
Tomatoes:					
fresh (table)	82.5	4.5	293.3	32.6	
sauce (frozen)	140.0	9.0	248.9	27.6	
jam	13.0	9.0	23.1	2.6	
pickled	15.1	9.0	26.8	3.0	
Leafy greens:					
frozen	15.4	5.0	49.3	5.5	
fresh	7.3	5.0	23.4	2.6	
Total	453.6		1,152.7	128.2	

So, if I can grow enough food to sustain me for six months in an area of 1,228 square feet (Table 5.3), then my garden would have to be twice that size (2,456 square feet) to grow a full year's worth. That sounds imposing until you realize it's less than a

Table 5-3. 2018, 2019, 2020 Garden Summary
Plots from 2018 and 2019, added to my 2020 garden, would theoretically feed me for 183 days, or six months.

Crop year	Weight Harvested lb.	Portions available	Days harvest would last at 9 portions per day	Area sq. ft.
2018-19	46.2	492.8	54.7	484
2020	452.3	1,152.8	128.1	744
Total	498.5	1,645.6	182.8	1,228

fourth the size of the average American lawn, which is 10,000 square feet. To feed myself for a year, I would need a sunny plot about 50' x 50', assuming no yield rate drop-offs from previous gardens. That would be over three times as large as my 2020 garden alone.

But that's with my 2019 corn spacing of 4 feet between rows and eight to ten inches between plants in a row, rather than the recommended standard of 2.5 feet between rows and 6 inches between plants in a row. Plus, you'll remember that in my 2020 garden I got rather low yields with the purple potatoes and Red

Kuri winter squash. By bringing yields for those two crops up to average, I should be able to do much better.

Following across Table 5-4, you can see that using the same plot sizes I'd previously used, but upgrading my technique to average spacing and yields, I could expect to get an added 144

Table 5-4. 2019 and 2020 yields vs. expected 2021 increases

Maximizing corn spacing and bringing potato and squash yields up to average would feed me for an additional 144 days.

	C^*	2019 and 2020 portion yields in my gardens $(D_1 = CH_1)$		2021 portion expected, based on average vegetable garden yields $(D_2 = CH_2)$		
		H_1 Harvest, lb.	D_1 Days harvest would last	H_2 Harvest, lb.	D_2 Days harvest would last	$D_2 - D_1$ Added days harvest would last
Corn (2019)	1.18	36.0	42.6	124	146.7	104.1
Potato (2020)	0.15	28.2	4.3	175	26.3	22.0
Squash (2020)	0.29	35.7	10.1	70	28.0	17.8
Totals		99.9	57.0	369	201.0	143.9

*Constant

days of sustenance compared to what I got in 2019-20 for those crops.

Putting this all together allows me to optimize the amount of space it would take for me to eat for a day, based on a hypothetical daily meal plan that could then be ramped up to a year. For this meal plan:

- There would be two calorie-rich items and one calorie-sparse item per meal.
- I would consume each vegetable only once per day, except for butter beans, eaten twice daily for protein.
- Meals would theoretically add up to about a pound of cooked food each for breakfast, lunch, and supper, which would equal 1,095 pounds per year—about average for an adult within a healthy weight range).

So, here's one way this meal plan could break out, using Table 5-5:

- **Breakfast:** corn (0.3) + butterbeans (0.4) + tomato (0.1) = **0.8 square feet**
- **Lunch:** potatoes (0.4) + squash (0.4) + green beans (1.0) = **1.8 square feet**
- **Supper:** greens (0.4) + sweet potato (0.5) + butterbeans (0.4) = **1.3 square feet**
- **Total: 4.1 square feet**

Of course, this is all just an example for the sake of illustration, as no one would want to eat the same breakfast, lunch, and supper every day for a year. This meal plan would require a total of 4.1 square feet of garden space per day. So, 365 days per year times 4.1 square feet per day equals 1,497 square feet for a year. That's 1/29ᵗʰ of an acre, versus the aforementioned three acres it takes to feed the average American for a year. It would be garden measuring about 39' x 39', compared to my 2020 garden of 24' x 31'.

Table 5-5. Area required per portion

It would theoretically take 4.1 square feet
of garden space per day to feed me.

Crop	Plot size, sq. ft.	Portions available	Sq. ft. per portion
Butter beans	48	108	0.4
Corn	352	1,077	0.3
Potatoes	84	240	0.4
Winter squash	84	224	0.4
Sweet potatoes	70	133	0.5
Green beans	168	161	1.0
Tomatoes	84	602	0.1
Greens	28	73	0.6
Butter beans	48	108	0.4
Total	966	2,726	4.1

Remember the 30' x 30' plot I cited in Chapter 3 that provides all the industrially-produced vegetables the average American eats per year, which would supply only 15 percent of their calorie needs? Compare that to a 39' x 39' plot that would provide all 100 percent of my calorie needs per year. Not that everyone needs to go the all-vegetable route; I don't intend to, for sure. I'm just showing what can be done.

So does this theoretical example reflect what's really possible, both on an individual scale as well as what could be ramped up nationwide? Could I *really* live from a garden measuring only 38' x 38'? I decided to find out by direct experience.

Garden Super-Size Me

Do you recall Morgan Spurlock's 2004 documentary, *Super-Size Me*, in which he ate nothing but McDonald's food every day for a month and recorded the disastrous effects on his body? Well, I decided to give my proposed home-grown food plan a similar test. Not to prove that a well-balanced diet of garden-grown veggies is generally much healthier than a solid McDonald's diet; most any nutritionist would agree that it is. Rather, my goal was to see if I could reasonably live for a month only on food from my garden, based on the meal plan in Table 5-5.

Like Spurlock, I first subjected myself to a thorough physical exam before I started, and then again after the month was over, just so I'd have some objective data on how it went. I recorded every ounce of each item I consumed, plus my subjective experiences, in a journal.

First, the basics: I ate only from my garden except for a few seasonings such as salt and pepper, herbs and spices, and a few shavings of fresh bacon (0.2 ounces per serving) to season beans and greens. Also, pepper vinegar, a sprinkling of parmesan cheese on tomato sauce, and butter and/or olive oil in which to sauté potatoes and sweet potatoes or to dribble over grits. In addition,

I allowed myself black and herb teas and exactly one cup of coffee with a sweet croissant, but no soft or alcoholic drinks, and no juices or processed drinks such as V-8 juice, energy drinks, or the like. In other words, 99.99 percent of what I ate came from the garden.

As I'm not a vegetarian, my first hurdle was to get over meat cravings. I was able to do that by making dishes as tasty as possible with the seasonings and, oddly, by treating my withdrawal symptoms with an occasional four to five teaspoons of salted almond butter between meals. After the first week or so I rarely needed even that. I also found that eating the pickled green tomatoes I made, whether with the salted almond butter or a meal, greatly helped soothe my need for a tasty treat.

The next challenge was the yearning for sweets. I'm not a big fan of heavy desserts; usually something like a single dark chocolate-covered piece of ginger or almond would be all I needed, but I did crave that. This is where my wife came to the rescue, as she made me some delicious tomato jam from my abundant supply of sweet tomatoes. It's something you never see here in the U.S., but it was common in her home country of Argentina, and she said it can also be found in Spain. So I'd just have a generous teaspoonful of that tasty jam once or twice daily. It also helped that big portions of sweet potatoes were on the menu every day.

In addition, I missed breads, biscuits, pasta, rice, and sandwiches, though not enough to have to invent something to counteract withdrawal symptoms.

Now, in spite of the fact that I ate only the eight vegetables in Tables 5-1 and 5-2, I enjoyed more variety than you might think. For example, tomatoes came in five options: fresh (red and orange), tomato sauce, pickled green tomatoes, and tomato jam.

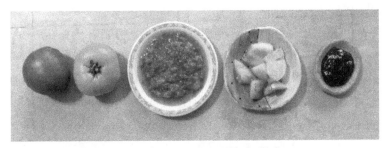

Tomatoes: fresh, sauce, pickled, and jam

I've been growing heirloom corn and making it into whole-grain grits and cornmeal for several years, so I had several colors and flavors to choose from: red (Bloody Butcher), blue and white (White Cherokee Eagle), and yellow (Northstine Dent).

Have you ever tried blue grits? Red grits? Or even yellow, which can also be thought of as polenta? I used all of those variations. Each retains its unique flavor and color—to varying degrees—when made into grits, dumplings, or hoecakes.

I also had butterbeans, cooked from either fresh or fresh frozen, or dried; all are the same variety of beans, but they deliver very different eating experiences. Likewise, green beans (Kentucky Wonders) were prepped from either fresh, frozen, or canned. Or harvested when the pods were dry, yielding shelled beans that taste a lot like pinto beans. I tried preparing all these options in a number of different ways, and combined them in a variety of permutations.

One thing I noticed after a couple weeks surprised me. Walking around in the grocery story with my wife (she was not on my garden diet), I suddenly became aware of feeling a little smug. Because I—unlike everyone else shopping for food—wasn't relying on someone else to keep me from starving. I was basically food self-sufficient, at least for a month, for the first time in my life. Quite a new and strange sensation, and distinctly empowering. Yes, I did use the seasonings I mentioned, but I knew that if I had to, I could even do without those. Or grow many of the herbs and seasonings myself, easily enough.

Also, when I made the lone exception to my garden diet by indulging in that sweet almond croissant with a cup of coffee to help my friend Mark celebrate passing his PhD defense, I had the oddest reaction. Although it tasted good, it felt vaguely artificial and unwelcome in my mouth, like some kind of superfluously-sweet fluff. That too surprised me, because I'm a big fan of good quality croissants. I suppose my tongue—and the rest of my body—was already getting used to a different physiological norm.

In any case, the food was delightfully savory, partly because I started getting creative. I really like pork or chicken sausage with breakfast, but since that was now off the menu, I decided to create my own sausage with the dry butterbeans. First I boiled them until they were soft, then mashed them up with diced red bell peppers from the garden and seasonings, made them into little patties, and sautéed them in an iron skillet in olive oil and butter. I call them Simon and Garfunkel sausages because of the parsley, sage, rosemary, and thyme I used to make them savory (along with salt, pepper, and that tiny bit of bacon shavings). They were so delicious I looked forward to having them every morning, especially since they wonderfully complemented the buttered grits and fresh tomato chunks or tomato pickles. What a treat!

Other innovations were tomato sauce over grits or winter squash, pickled tomatoes with almost everything, and butter-sautéed, diced purple potatoes that had been pre-boiled. Of course, the harvest from my 2020 garden, even when augmented by leftover beans and corn from previous gardens, wouldn't last a whole year, so I'm once again buying food in the grocery store. Still, it will be interesting to see what the longer-term effects will be. I'm already eating a lot more vegetables than I used to, and also those Simon and Garfunkel butter bean sausages.

At end of the month, I found that although my energy level was good throughout, I had lost three pounds. I'm guessing my body found it quite a shock to suddenly be deprived of meat, although a two percent weight drop over 30 days isn't too concerning. My follow-up physical exam revealed that my blood pressure, already in the healthy range when I started at 136/70, was now 108/50. The nurse had no explanation, but wasn't worried; evidently blood pressure can vary that much from one day to the next, or even within a day. Also, my level of vitamin B12 had decreased a little, not surprising in view of having almost no meat or dairy for a month. My hemoglobin dropped slightly and my iron went up a bit, and my PSA was a tad high. None of which was particularly concerning to the nurse, as all were close to norms. Most significantly, my cholesterol had dropped from 230 to 216. Since I'd had slightly high cholesterol for years, the nurse viewed that as an encouraging outcome.

Having proven that I can subsist on my own garden food for a month, the next step would be to extend it to a year. But to do that, I should first reveal what I actually ate during that month, just going by what felt right according to taste and satisfaction. As I mentioned in my proposed meal plan (Table 5-5), I had intended to have daily one portion each of corn, winter squash, potatoes, sweet potatoes, tomatoes, leafy greens, and green beans, plus two portions of butter beans. That is, three portions per meal, in various permutations. However, as indicated in Table 5-6, I ended up having about nine times as many portions of corn as winter squash, with a range of consumption rates between those extremes for the other veggies. I'd also intended to consume calorie-rich to calorie-sparse portions at a ratio of 2 to 1, but the actual ratio came out to about 2.4 to 1. In general, I found that I had to eat a *lot* of calorie-rich veggies just to maintain my weight (which I tracked all along). This may be potentially good news for people who want to lose weight, especially if, unlike me, they favor calorie-sparse options.

Table 5-6. Monthly and Projected Yearly Area Usage

Based on the rates at which I consumed eight vegetables over a month, I would need 1,351 square feet to provide all my food for a year—a garden about 37' x 37'.

Crop	Portions consumed per month	Portions consumed per year	Sq. ft. per portion	Sq. ft. per yr. required
Corn	90	1,080	0.3	324.0
Butter beans	66	792	0.4	316.8
Tomatoes	56	672	0.1	67.2
Potatoes	29	348	0.4	139.2
Leafy greens	25	300	0.6	180.0
Sweet potatoes	24	288	0.5	144.0
Green beans	11	132	1.0	132.0
Winter squash	10	120	0.4	48.0
Total	311	3,732	3,732	1,351.2

Surprisingly, based on the record of what I actually ate for a month, and the area it would take to grow each vegetable for a year, it would require only 1,351 square feet, or a plot 34' x 40', to grow a year's worth of food. That's over 1,000 square feet less than the 2,456 square feet I would have needed based on my 2018 and 2019 corn and bean plots plus the entire 2020 garden. And it's just a little less than the 1,497 square feet predicted from Table 5.5. That's encouraging. I'm sure the low figure is due to more efficient spacing as well as the fact that I ate so much corn (mostly in the form of grits), and butterbeans, both of which require the least amount of area per harvested calorie to grow, as you'll see in Chapter 8. I'm not sure I'd eat like that over a year, so the size of my 2021 garden is 1,400 square feet, or 35' x 40', just to have a little extra space to try out a greater variety of vegetables.

That's still a very manageable garden plot. As of the end of November, I had already prepped the needed 218 feet of new turf, spading it 8 inches deep and 16 inches wide, and leaving two-foot-wide grass aisles between beds. It took me only 15 minutes to dig seven feet of row per day, or about a month to do the whole thing, plus a day or two off from time to time due to inclement weather. In the spring, I'll just mix in a little compost, plant the crops, and add leaves I raked up this fall for mulch. Then I'll use the grass clippings I will have gathered from spring mowing for additional mulch. That will help to keep moisture in the soil and weeds down around the plants. Easy. I've done it all before. Fifteen to thirty minutes max of "work" per day, or three-and-a-half hours per week to feed myself for a year. Pretty close to the average four hours a week that gardeners spend growing things. And for me, it is more like enjoyable relief from clacking away on a keyboard than work.

Meanwhile, this year's (2020) garden didn't end with the close of summer. During the first week of September, I transplanted seedlings of kale, chard, and other greens to one of the beds where I'd harvested potatoes. Six weeks later, those greens reached harvestable size, and I've already gotten a number of meals' worth as of mid-December. So far, they've stayed alive and healthy down to 13°F, as they're winter-hardy. To extend this harvest of fresh, living produce even longer—possibly through a winter that will surely get down to well below zero—I made protective, plastic-covered elongated boxes to cover them when it gets really cold. It's a nice new garden project, and it will be interesting to see how long they keep the greens alive.

I designed the boxes so that, while firmly attached to the ground at the back corners, I can leave the greens completely exposed. I can also swing the boxes up to a tilt to partly cover the plants, or completely cover them when it gets down to 20 degrees or lower.

I also left some of the greens with no cover at all, just as a control to see how much longer the covers extend my winter harvest. As a fierce winter storm blew my cold frames half a block away several years ago, these boxes are anchored not only at the back corners but are also secured at the front corners when closed, and otherwise strongly tethered at each of the other two positions. As well, I made them to withstand blizzards, ice storms, heavy snow, windstorms, and whatever else the howling winter might throw at them.

I've thus embarked on succession planting, something I had never tried before. If this little experiment in winter greens is successful, I'll for sure try out more of the same in the future, which will make my garden even more productive than that depicted in Table 5-6. That's the creative fun of gardening— always more interesting things to try out next.

So what does it all mean, this 30-day garden diet experiment, supplied by some of the produce from of my 2018, 2019, and 2020 gardens? Simply that—to reiterate my statement of purpose at the end of Chapter 1—given very few resources, a little know-how, and a pace that works for you, you can be food self-sufficient, or largely so, with a moderate amount of enjoyable effort.

6

Me? Start a garden?
I Don't Have the . . .

I understand.

The prospect of growing a vegetable garden, even a small one, can be intimidating if you've never done it before, or at most have only a potted tomato plant on your patio. Just the thought of digging in the dirt, sweating in the broiling sun while your back and knees are aching and ants are crawling up your shorts might be enough to send you scurrying back to your comfy couch and the TV remote.

Or maybe it's just too scary. One woman I was teaching how to garden actually screamed at the sight of a big, wriggling earthworm I held up in my hand for her to inspect, thinking she would be impressed at this living evidence of healthy soil in her yard. However, she overcame her initial trepidations and was willing to give it a go, slimy worm from hell or not. So I give her all the credit in the world.

Reasons not to garden are many and may seem convincing, but ultimately they're not really valid once you look more closely at them, at least not for most people. So let's see if we can de-fang them.

Time

I just don't have the time. Lord knows, with a full-time job, kids to raise, and housework, which my wife hardly ever helps me with, there's just no way I have the time to grow a garden.

Time is a funny thing. People tend to think about it like death and taxes. Sixty minutes per hour, twenty-four hours a day, seven days a week—nothing you can do about that. But the odd thing is, the less time you think you have, the less you have. For example, I have a professor friend who once complained to me about the "time famine." Simply not enough time to do what he wanted and needed to do, not even close. Contrast that with my grandmother, whose husband died from leukemia when he was 45, leaving her, at age 43, with three kids to take care of, during World War II. Her resilient, wise attitude, which she later emphasized to us grandchildren many times over, was, "You always have time to do what you want to do."

That philosophy of time served her well as she moved on with her life, putting all three of those kids through college. Without remarrying. Working as a mill hand. In a non-unionized cotton mill. In the South. Matter of fact, it was the very mill portrayed in the 1979 movie, *Norma Rae*, starring Sally Field. In further point of fact, my grandmother knew the real-life Norma Rae, who struggled against all odds to unionize that cotton mill. Anyway, the point is that Grandma had all kinds of challenging life circumstances lined up against her, yet still firmly believed she had all the time she needed to do anything she wanted to. Straight out simple, with no conditions, no ifs, ands, or buts. As opposed to my tenured college professor friend in a cushy, well-paid office job, who had far more life circumstances lined up in his favor, convinced that time was disappearing into the famine.

So, which philosophy of time do you think would serve you better as you ponder whether you have the time to put in a vegetable garden? Especially when the average American spends about four hours a day watching TV, and three and a half on digital media. (But wait, that's almost eight hours a day. How is there ever time to earn a living? Oh, I know. People "save" time by watching TV and keeping up with social media at the same time. Hmmm ... could all that ~~saved~~ lost TV/digital time be contributing to the time famine?)

Now here's an encouraging fact to consider. Did you know that people who garden spend only about four hours a week at it? Which is about what I spend. So if you're still overwhelmed by the I-don't-have-the-time concern, do you think maybe, just maybe, it might be *time* to throw it out?

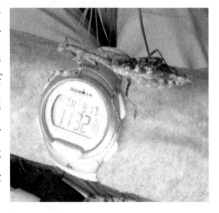

Space

Okay, I win on this one for sure. I don't even have a yard. So I can't have a garden. Period.

It's indeed unfortunate if you don't have a yard, although if you're reading this book it's not likely to be an insurmountable obstacle. Do you have a sunny porch or patio, even a small one? Even though you couldn't grow all that much food on it, a container pot with a tomato plant or a potato "tower" could still give you the empowering experience of growing at least some of your own food. How about wall brackets and trellises, window boxes, space for dwarf varieties, and wooden pallets and boxes? They also can host growing things.

Or, have you checked to see if there is a community garden in your area that provides individual plots for people? If not, maybe your best bet is to get your fresh food from one of the other local options, such as farmers markets, CSAs, urban farms, and the like. Or even, to partner up with someone and start up some kind of gardening venture that doesn't yet exist in your neighborhood. After all, you have the time to do it if it's something you really want to do. And, you can most likely spare a little of your TV/digital time without losing anything of value.

On the other hand, if you're one of the 102 million Americans who have a lawn, chances are you won't be able to glom onto this reason for not gardening. Unless, say, your lawn gets less than eight hours of direct sunshine a day, in which case see if a neighbor with a sun-splashed lawn has a spot she's willing to share. Or go the community garden route. But if you do have a sunny area and are still doubtful about starting up a garden, you may want to fish for a more promising reason among the other wonderful options below. There's still a pretty fair number to pick and choose from.

Water

We don't get much rain where I live, and I don't look forward to setting up a watering system, much less paying for the cost of getting and the trouble of running it. Water is expensive, dude.

One, the average size of an American lawn is 10,000 square feet, whereas a potentially profitable 300 sq. ft. vegetable garden (15' x 20') is much smaller. Two, it costs much more to water the average lawn than a small- to medium-sized garden, so if your lawn is not dried up and brown, chances are you can afford to water a garden. Especially since grass is the largest irrigated crop in the nation.

Vegetables do need to be well-watered. In many regions, rain will take care of it, but if you do need to water, a single lawn sprinkler will cover a 15' x 20' plot nicely. Or, if you want to get much more efficient, drip irrigation is the way to go, especially if your garden is larger than 300 sq. ft. As with many other garden needs, once you make that initial investment (which will vary depending on the size of your garden), it becomes another fixed-cost implement you can use year after year. In almost all scenarios it would pay for itself pretty quickly in profits.

Aptitude

Well, look, I'm just one of those people who doesn't have a green thumb. Plants don't like me. Every plant I touch dies. It's hopeless.

Oh, dear, I am *so* sorry to hear that you've come down with PAGA. I know that Pro-Active Gardening Aversion can strike anyone, at any age, without warning. Yet every single human being has a natural affinity for plants, and nature in general; it's called biophilia. The perceived lack thereof, including Woody Allen's perception that "Nature and I are two," is just that—a notion not rooted in the fertile soil of fact (sorry, Woody). Of course, some people are allergic to plants, but they're few. And even they have an affinity for plants; they just can't physically interact with them. So fine, someone else has to grow their food. But unless you have such allergies, you can't credibly beg out of starting a garden on the premise that plants hate you.

Know-How

Okay, let's say I have the time, space, water, aptitude, and have gotten over the idea that I scare plants to death. I still don't have any basic knowledge of gardening, and I really don't want to take a course on the subject. Or worse, read a book on it. Because I don't read books.

No problem, because you don't have to become a gardening maestro to grow your first garden. In fact, unless you're the super-strong, gung-hoe type, already outdoorsy hale-and-hearty, or have an experienced gardener friend to advise you every step of the way, I recommend that you start out small and simple. That is, in such a way that it doesn't require much more skill than digging a hole in the ground with a spade, fluffing the soil up a little while mixing in a little compost, and planting some seeds. If that's too much work or more than you can physically handle, call in Super Teen-Age Girl. Or the Teen-Age Boy version thereof. Don't worry, he's just as willing and capable. Or maybe you're lucky enough to still be a teenager yourself. Only thing is, then you'd have even less reason to beg off gardening.

Maybe your first garden is a only a few feet square. You saw in Chapter 1 how incredibly much food you can produce in a 27' x 31' plot. The point is, just get started. I'll give you a few recommendations in the next chapter, but allow yourself to grow little by little, nurturing yourself with knowledge acquired here and there as you go about nurturing your plants. Because, in a very real sense, your plants grow you just as much as you grow them. Or to put it another way, they grow on you (not literally, of course). That's an empowering—and simultaneously concern-easing—way to think about it.

Strength

I'm just not the strongest or most able person to be digging or crawling around on my hands and knees pulling weeds.

Scanning through the internet, I see some people claiming that gardening is physically demanding, hard work, while others insist it's quite easy. My own experience is definitely in the latter category. Nonetheless, I can see how, if someone is used to a mostly sedentary life, starting to indiscriminately flail about with a shovel could be exhausting. So just start small and gentle. If you are physically impaired, look for a little help from a neighborhood friend or teenager. Or put an ad on your community bulletin board asking for volunteer help, or even offering to pay for a little gardening assistance. You'll probably be surprised at how happy people are to help you, and the money you save will cover the ad, for sure. Not to mention, you'll likely find that you'll be doing more to help your helper than you ever imagined.

Self-Confidence

The whole thing is just too much. I'd probably either make a mess of it, lose interest after spending a bunch of money, or burn out with nothing to show for it. Worse, my obnoxious neighbor would then lean over the fence and laugh at me. "Hey, farmer Bob [or Sue], didn't quite work out, huh? Ha ha. Looks like it's back to the couch for you."

This is the third of the I-simply-don't-have-it-in-me concerns. So, here's the prescription for maximizing your chances of success if you're still self-dubious. Again, keep your gardening venture small to begin with. Then, plant only the very easiest things to take care of, maybe just tomatoes, bell peppers, and winter squash, or whatever most appeals to you. Only then should you work your way up to more ambitious crops. And don't worry about the snarky neighbor, it's not worth it. Because who knows? If you're determined enough to succeed you just might get to enjoy the perverse but benign satisfaction of offering him a big, plump, luscious tomato right off your very first plant. Hah!

Tools

I don't have the tools I'd need for gardening. And don't I have to get some kind of tractor or rototiller to prep the soil? I can't afford that.

Let's face it: the biggest barrier to growing a garden is often, well, just starting. That includes initial investments, which some studies present as what you need to subtract from your first year's efforts to see if you come out ahead. Financial profit doesn't always happen at first, and even if you do get one, it often doesn't look very impressive. However, once you have garden tools, maybe a 2' high chicken wire fence to keep out rabbits, and have done your initial cultivation of the soil, you don't need to begin all over again each year from scratch. And yes, I'm aware that a 2' high fence won't keep out deer, if that's your worry. So just install a higher fence; it's not that expensive.

Assuming you do start simple and can get someone to demonstrate the basics of how to use it, the only tool you really need at first is a sturdy, D-handle shovel about three and a half feet long with a flat, reasonably sharp, hard-steel blade no wider than about 8". That's all I needed, spading about fifteen minutes every day or so over a few weeks, to turn and fluff up the soil for my first Midwest 25' x 50'garden, right here in heavy-clay soil Iowa. If you start with a plot about 15' x 20', which I recommend for a newbie, it would take even less time and effort. Especially if, like me, you only spade 16'-wide beds for planting, leaving 2' of lawn between beds as a grassy walking aisle. So unless you can't afford to buy and are unable to borrow a spade, lack of tools is not really a deal-killer. If you don't already know how to properly use a spade, to avoid putting undue strain on your back or arms, it's essential to get someone to show you how. It's really not difficult once you get the hang of it.

Later, yeah, you might benefit from having a good rototiller. Or you might want to hire someone to plow up a small portion of your lawn to save you the effort of spading it. Maybe at some point you'd want to add a hoe and a rake. I have those, and a few other hand tools, but I only use them occasionally.

Seeds

I've read that seed companies have seen sales go through the roof, and I've had friends tell me that they weren't even able to get the more popular seeds at all.

All of that was true from about mid-February to mid-May, 2020, because the seed companies, like everyone else except for a few public health experts, didn't see this pandemic coming. Seeds, sales of which increased tenfold this spring[1], were in such short supply it was called the toilet paper of the gardening world.

However, the merchants of seed hope seem to have recovered, as by July I was getting promotions from companies that I couldn't get some seed varieties from in March. I suspect, after talking to the CEO of one of the largest garden seed companies, that they'll be well prepared for even more intense demand for the 2021 planting season. Still, it wouldn't hurt to get your seeds as soon as possible, as another big run on them was gearing up already in February 2021.

As for cost, most varieties you'd need for a start-up garden are around $3 a packet, and you wouldn't need many of them. Regarding your investment, remember (from Chapter 2) that for a $4 packet of heirloom corn seed I grew $450 worth of corn on the little plot in my 2018 garden, and two packets could have brought a $1,060 profit from an even smaller plot with more efficient, standard spacing for corn. Just say'n.

Permission

My significant other would never let me do this, protesting that I have more important things to do, like making more money to buy food by working harder or longer at my job. Besides, we have a ban on growing a garden on our lawn. Blemishes the looks of the neighborhood and reduces the value of the house, etc.

In most places permission isn't a problem, especially if your garden is in your back yard. But if you live in a neighborhood with a homeowner association, it may be, so check to see what kind of regulations apply to you. If you're prohibited from using any part of your lawn for a garden, you may want to refer to *Biting the Hand That Feeds You*, by Baylen J. Linekin.[2] He has a lot of suggestions. As for getting permission from your significant other, just reiterate all the individual benefits, including saving money on groceries, that could come from a garden. Or have him or her read this book. Who knows, maybe they'll even get inspired by the bigger-picture reasons for starting up a garden. Like the potentially satisfying prospect of helping to cool the planet or out-doing—in terms of yield rate—industrial agriculture.

7

Getting Started

Gardening strategies

As this book is more about making the case for starting (or expanding) a vegetable garden than a how-to on the subject, I'll just hit some highlights of the gardening process itself.

There are many styles and methods of home vegetable gardening, so how do you know which is the best? To tell the truth, I'm not sure it matters all that much. People get lush, highly productive home vegetable gardens using a wide variety of approaches, each advocate swearing by their favorite. Some of the more common, with a variety of different angles, are (in no particular order):

More or Less Conventional

- *The Four-Season Harvest*—Elliott Coleman

  With the likes of plastic covered low- and high- hoop tunnels, Coleman extends production of fresh vegetables from spring and summer gardening—for which he has well thought out and tried out methods aplenty—right through the fall and winter, even where he lives in Maine.

- *Biointensive*—John Jeavons

  Sometimes called Grow Biointensive, this method combines close inter-planting with an all-out effort to improve soil fertility by double-digging, intelligent use of water, and incorporating copious amounts of compost into the soil. It can build fertile soil much deeper and faster than nature does it.

- *Gardening Without Work*—Ruth Stout

  The book's subtitle says it all: *For the Aging, Busy, and Indolent*. The idea is to grow fresh fruits and vegetables without a spade, hoe, or plow, and without worrying about irrigation, spraying, cover crops, weeding, cultivating, or even building a compost pile.

- *Gardening When It Counts* –Steve Solomon

  This approach helps readers to cope with difficult times by raising a family garden with just four hand tools and little or no irrigation and electricity. It brings back sustainable systems common before the 1970s but now largely forgotten.

- *Raised Bed Gardening for Beginners*—Tammy Wylie

  Reasons for using raised beds include less bending because of the elevated ground level, better soil drainage, quicker soil warming in the spring, grass control, and the option to add better quality soil over your foundation if all you have is rocky dirt or subsoil.

- *The Autopilot Garden*—Luke Marion

  The key idea here is to organize your garden so well that once you've established well thought out systems for handling cultivation, planting, weeding, water, and space, it will run on for the rest of the season on autopilot, saving you time and hassle.

- *Permaculture*—Bill Mollison and David Holmgren

  Permaculture is a holistic gardening design system that draws on the way natural ecosystems work. It's governed by a set of 12 principles such as catch and store energy, value and use diversity, produce no waste, integrate rather than segregate, and use small and slow solutions.

More on the alternative side

- *Biodynamics*—Rudolf Steiner

  In addition to being a detailed gardening strategy, biodynamics was the first of the organic agricultural movements. Although it uses sound ecological concepts, especially regarding soil fertility, it also incorporates elements such as observation of lunar phases and planetary cycles, incantations, and ritual substances.

- *Perelandra*—Machaelle Small Wright

  This is an esoteric system of gardening that Wright says was taught to her by nature itself, and hence "thumbs its nose" at tradition and logic. It is gardening as a metaphor for life, she says, and will change the way you do everything else in your life.

- *Findhorn*—the Findhorn Community

  Findhorn began with Peter Caddy, who, during a period of unemployment starting in 1962, began to experiment with organic gardening in rocky soil in Findhorn, Scotland. His results, produced in part by communication with natural spirits, were so remarkable they eventually attracted national attention and inspired an ongoing gardening and spiritual community.

Going all out

- *Backyard homesteading—Lisa Lombardo, David Toht, Carleen Madigan, Ron and Johanna Melchiore, and others*

  The typical goal of this route is for a family to be largely or totally off the grid self-sufficient. It tends to cover not only food but also water, electricity, heating, cooling, and waste disposal needs, as well as animal care and how to build out the required physical infrastructure. Clearly more ambitious than the typical home garden, but with a lot of useful how-to information nonetheless.

Just reading over these summary descriptions, even though I wrote them myself and have been gardening off and (mostly) on for about 60 years, makes me want to try all of them. There are many more approaches, including a fair number of online starter "kits" or automated, preplanned systems that aim to help you start and maintain a vegetable garden.

All of these methods reflect the art and science of dedicated, expert gardeners who have put decades of heart and soul into their work. You can benefit more than you can imagine from any of them. I urge you to check through them and see which appeals the most to you. Or maybe you'll decide to combine, adopting practices from a variety of approaches, as I have.

Regenerative

I'd be remiss if I didn't mention the fact that these days "regenerative" is replacing organic and sustainable as the latest hot concept for all that's desirable in the realm of growing food and organizing life in general. Ethan Soloviev describes the difference in terms of paradigms: regenerative focuses on "evolve capacity" (continuous development of complementary ecological and human processes), whereas organic mainly aims to "do no harm" (no chemical pesticides, fertilizers, GMOs, etc.). Regenerative is more holistic, inclusive, and expansive than organic, especially in the realms of social justice and cultural equity. For instance, it would be possible to have a certified organic farm that's oppressive to workers. Not so with regenerative. Still, organic and regenerative practices do complement one another, and both have positive impacts on the land, food, and human health.

On the other hand, both are also typically applied primarily to farms. So here is how a combination of organic *and* regenerative would play out in home gardens or community garden plots.

Increasing biodiversity

Replacing a patch of lawn with a variety of vegetables obviously increases plant diversity (unless you start with an especially weedy lawn). It also greatly increases the diversity of soil organisms that will go on to improve soil health. In addition, many seed companies offer packets of a variety of seeds you can disperse around or in your garden to grow plants that encourage birds, beneficial predator insects, and pollinators.

Improving watersheds

It's important to use water wisely, whether it comes from your house, a well, or precipitation. That means increasing organic matter in your soil with compost and using a substantial cover of mulch, both of which increase soil water retention. That, in turn, reduces the need to draw on your house water supply in times of drought, or in places that are virtually always short on water, such as much of the American West and Southwest. If you do have to depend on city water, use drip irrigation rather than lawn sprinklers, thereby easing the pull on watersheds. You might even consider something more ambitious, such as diverting rainwater from your roof down the gutter and into a water barrel, which could then gravity-feed your nearby garden. Just one possibility.

Enriching the soil

Again, good quality compost and organic fertilizers are a must. By enriching, I mean supplying the soil with the organic matter and minerals it needs to foster the diversity of soil organisms that make nutrients available to plant roots. Sure, nitrogen is nitrogen, whether it's in compost or a chemical fertilizer. But feeding the soil with a concentrated fertilizer like pure, granulated NPK (nitrogen, phosphorus, and potassium) is like dumping a spoonful of pure, granulated sugar into your mouth. The NPK produces as much damaging shock to the living system of the soil as the sugar does to the living system of your mouth. That's why compost is as delicious to the soil organisms as a juicy, ripe peach is to your tongue. Both artificially concentrated and naturally complex fertilizers provide necessary nutrients, but compost does it gently, in ways that enhance and enrich the soil rather than shock and degrade it. In addition, good quality compost has far more nutrients than pure NPK.

Capturing carbon

All green plants capture carbon during photosynthesis, but what's often meant by this term is artificially removing it from the atmosphere and dumping it deep into the earth. It also refers to the fact that plants not only capture carbon, they sequester it in the "soil bank," through root exudates, much like the way people deposit money in their bank. To continue the analogy, money in a regular bank can be invested in the health and wealth of the community, just as carbon deposited into the soil is an investment in the health of the soil and anything growing in it. By using high inputs such as chemical fertilizers and soil pesticides, industrial agriculture has brought about the removal of more soil carbon—75% of it so far—than it's deposited.

By using compost and natural mulch you can regenerate healthy soil that may have been largely degraded by decades of synthetic chemical use. In fact, you can even increase it beyond what nature alone would do. In this way, you're serving as an agent of nature by increasing the depth and well-being of your topsoil much faster than would happen if left to natural processes.

And not just for your garden alone. If replicated on a large scale, home gardens, along with regenerative local food systems, would greatly help to remove excess carbon from the atmosphere and stash it in the soil, as noted in Chapter 3. That, in turn, would reduce global warming substantially. In fact, on a global scale agriculture could do much to help return the amount of atmospheric carbon to pre-industrial levels simply by using regenerative practices that result in net sequestration in the soil.

Increasing yield

From the evidence and examples I've provided so far, and there are more in Chapter 8, it's clear that when considered at a whole system level, regenerative home gardens and local food systems would average more food per acre and waste far less than the industrial system. And that's not even accounting for the enormous external costs of the current system, discussed in Chapter 6.

Enhancing ecological services

Ecological services are those natural processes that provide us with the basics we need to live. For example, photosynthesis gives us all the oxygen we breathe and all the food (directly or indirectly) we eat. Another example is the hydrological cycle, recycling water from the ocean to land through evaporation and the wind, which is an ecological service in itself. Other services include the cooling action of plants, both by shading and evapotranspiration, and the decomposition of organic matter by bacteria and fungi to the minerals plants need to grow.

The home gardener can participate in the delivery of nature's ecological services by aiding and abetting them. For instance, you can help regenerate nature's provision of organic matter by feeding kitchen scraps, yard wastes, and leftover plant matter from your garden to the decomposer microbes in a compost heap. Including non-food plants in your garden that attract birds, pollinators, and other beneficial insects is another example. Although most natural gardening philosophies seek to make use of ecological services, permaculture, biointensive, and all of the alternative approaches make even more focused efforts to maximize them, very much in the vein of regenerative food production.

Producing more nutrient-dense food

This concept was introduced in Chapter 2, in the context of retaining higher levels of vitamins and minerals in heirloom, landrace, and other crop plants that have not been subjected to decades of breeding primarily for industrial harvest, storage, and long-distance shipping. Not to mention retaining and even increasing soil nutrition, which then improves human nutrition.

Improving communities

Even if you have an individual garden, you get more out of it when you have neighbors who also garden. Swap gardening techniques, inside knowledge of the tastiest varieties, tips learned from successes and failures, and even the vegetables themselves. Hey, I'll trade you a few of my golden beets for some of your luscious-looking spinach. Deal?

How I did it

As for myself, I just learned as I went, starting at about age twelve. I picked up a few ideas from my dad and have been improving and improvising my technique ever since. Sometimes years would go by when I didn't have a full garden as I got busy being a sailor, student, researcher, or professor. But I always

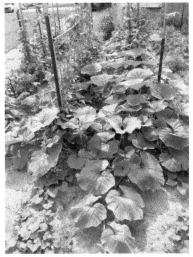

came back to it when a place to dig up a plot of soil became available. For the last 17 years I've had a plot of variable size next to the apartment building where I live.

How have I done on my latest efforts? Well enough so that—based on my yields of corn, beans, and winter squash—I calculated that I'd

The Summer Garden

need only a tenth of an acre to meet my food needs for a year. That's equal to a fifth of the world average for the amount of land needed to feed one per person per year (Americans need much more, as we saw with the 3-acre per capita average). And that was before I became much more efficient, producing higher yields in less space.

Surprising, when you consider that I:

- Used only a shovel (mostly), hoe, and rake
- Averaged only about 15-30 minutes per day hand-

turning the soil in the spring, and fertilizing, weeding, watering, and mulching over the summer

- Was gardening in topsoil from who knows where that was dumped there after extensive landscaping on the site
- Didn't use any chemical fertilizers or pesticides
- Did all this while holding down a demanding full-time job

The point is, you don't need to be a gardening fanatic, working the land from dawn to dusk by the proverbial sweat of your brow, to grow an impressive amount of food on a small amount of land—even if you're only using hand tools.

Did I have setbacks? Of course I did, and still do. Following various experiences with destruction, I have had to figure out simple, non-toxic, animal- and ecologically friendly ways to protect my crops from chipmunks, crows and other birds, deer, groundhogs, rabbits, insects, voles, raccoons, violent summer storms, and droughts. These efforts required a wheelbarrow, fences, humane traps or other forms of deterrence, organic insect control, physical support for pole beans, and drip irrigation. All of this was implemented little by little over the years, so it wasn't nearly as substantial as it might appear here.

Beginning from zero experience

If you're absolutely new to gardening, start with the simple and small, and build from there with inspiration, comfort, and fun as your primary motivators. You won't stay at it for long if it's not enjoyable and fulfilling.

Yes, a rototiller can greatly reduce the cultivation labor, but it's not necessary if you're of sound body, average strength, and can learn a little about how to properly handle a shovel, hoe, and rake.

It's important to remember that you need a spot with at least eight hours of direct sunlight. Ten is better. Then, choose a plot of soil—whether it's your back yard, an empty lot in a city (for which you will need to get permission), or soil in some kind of container, such as a pot on a patio or a raised bed on a rooftop.

As for storage, dried corn, beans, winter squash, and sweet potatoes can be stored in a cool, dry place. Irish potatoes need to be stored in a cool, dark, humid, and well-ventilated place such as a damp basement. Of course, home canning and/or freezing will extend your range of vegetable choices. I grow Brandywine tomatoes that I use along with onions, green peppers, and celery to make single-serving portions of tomato sauce, which I freeze in small plastic bags. I then use those throughout the cold months for spaghetti sauce, chili, lasagna, etc. Drying is also an option if you have a countertop dehydrator or live in a climate arid enough to dry things in the sun.

What to grow—maximizing nutrition, yield, and storage ease

My goal this year (2021) was to grow what I thought would help tide me over if there did turn out to be some kind of food shortage or disruption because of the pandemic. That's why I focused on selections from what I call the Terrific Ten: corn, dry beans, winter squash, potatoes, sweet potatoes, carrots, green (snap) beans, tomatoes, bell peppers, and leafy greens. Of those, in 2020 I grew all but corn and carrots. I'm also growing okra.

That's not to say that many other of your favorite veggies won't do; I just chose these as the most important in addressing immediate needs of calories and nutrients to support a robust, healthy diet.

Better taste is the most common reason for growing heirloom varieties, according to Solomon[1] as well as the National Garden Association. And although tastes vary, I've found that the higher the nutrient content, including oils and proteins as well as vitamins, minerals, antioxidants, the more flavorful a vegetable is. Makes sense, because it's those kinds of nutrients that the taste buds especially pick up on, as opposed to the equally necessary but not as tasty starch. The natural sugar in sweet fruits and vegetables is not only tasty but also calorie-rich.

What follows are my recommendations for what to grow in a subsistence garden packed with the most appropriate vegetables to provide you with nutritious food, ideally for a year. (For a portion-based approach, refer back to Chapter 5.) It's important to plant about twice as much calorie-dense veggies (corn, potatoes, winter squash, beans, and sweet potatoes) as the calorie-sparse (tomatoes, carrots, greens, sweet peppers, and green beans). It's surprising how often garden plans, on balance, seem to favor nutritious but watery vegetables over calorie-dense types.

Primarily for calories, but also nutritious

Corn

You've already heard me rave about Bloody Butcher, the variety of red heirloom corn that yielded well for me. Evidently it's also quite nutritious, as it's very similar to Floriani Red, the variety used in the nutrient study mentioned in Chapter 2.

Bear in mind that I'm talking about dent or flint corn that's dried for producing grits and cornmeal, simply because leaving the corn on the plant until it dries gives it more time to accumulate calories and nutrients. I also love fresh sweet corn, but I rely on the local farmers market for that. My reason is that to grow corn you need a minimum of four 10' rows side by side for effective pollination, and that would produce far more sweet corn than I would eat. Of course, I could just pick some of my heirloom corn early for fresh eating, or can or freeze it. But I prefer to dry and store it until I'm ready to whip up a serving of grits, or cornmeal for dumplings.

Another variety that's apparently tasty and nutritious, but not as high-yielding, is New England Eight Row Flint corn. And then there's Hopi Blue, with 30% higher protein than conventional dent corns. There are endless varieties of modern and age-old heirloom sweet, flint, dent, and flour corn, and of course popcorn; the ones I mention are a good place to start to get the most nutrition bang for your buck. Or to put it more aptly, energy for your effort. Or taste for your toil? Okay, okay, I'll stop there, I promise.

Potatoes

Spuds tend to get a bad rap because they're perceived as being nothing but starch and usually eaten in the form of French fries or potato chips loaded with fat and salt. And it's true that peeled, white-fleshed russet potatoes, boiled or fried, are a bland feast of starch. But that's not the kind of potatoes I recommend— although I have to say, Yukon Golds aren't half bad.

Rather, I'd like to put in a word for my favorite: all purple (or all blue) potatoes. That is, those with purple flesh, as opposed to ones that have purple skins only. Eaten with the skin, all purples are a surprisingly tasty and a nutritious source of fiber, manganese, copper, iron, potassium, vitamin B6, vitamin C, and protein.

Protein? Potatoes?! That's right, potatoes have more protein per pound than any other vegetable. That's why, in the 1800s in Ireland, poor people could get most of their protein needs from potatoes. Of course, they had to eat a heck of a lot of potatoes, but that's exactly what they did. It was a subsistence food. When the potato crop failed due to Late Blight in the 1840s, many Irish people died (about a million) or emigrated (another million). However, the real reason for the famine was that the Irish and

British governments refused to help, even though they were both exporting food at that time.

Still not convinced about the protein? Then wrap your mind around this: by dry weight, potatoes contain up to 11% protein, which equals the protein content of human breast milk.[2]

As for starch, purple potatoes have a glycemic index of 77, compared to yellow potatoes of 81, and white potatoes of 93.[3] Glycemic index is a measure of the extent to which a food increases blood sugar, with lower values considered healthier than higher values. The all-purples also have two to three times more health-promoting antioxidants than large, white potatoes, and may improve blood pressure and reduce cancer risk.[4]

In addition to their nutritional value, I think their rich, almost buttery taste is just much more flavorful than most white- or yellow-fleshed potatoes. Some varieties of all purple are higher yielding than others, so you'll want to research what grows best in your area. If you go for yield above all, the white- and yellow-fleshed varieties will probably give you more pounds per plant. At least, that's been my experience. So you have to decide whether it's worth it to plant more of an all-purple variety to get the total amount you want. I say it is, and that's what I usually do. As you'll certainly find out, if you haven't already, gardening is full of such decisions.

Winter squash

Varieties of winter squash number in the scores if not hundreds, but the one you typically hear about first and foremost is butternut. It's sweet and tasty, easy to grow because it's resistant to squash vine borer, and is a reasonably good producer. It retains its moisture better than most others when baked, and lasts months while not occupying much storage room. That's because its seed cavity is small, unlike pumpkins and many others with big cavities. The vines require more space than most other varieties, and butternuts don't last in storage quite as long as some, but otherwise you can't go wrong with them.

As for nutrition, acorn squash appears to come out on top, although all deep yellow- or orange-fleshed winter squashes, including Butternut, Delicata, Hubbard, and Buttercup, are rich in nutrients—especially carotenes, vitamin C, fiber and antioxidants. It's hard to quantify yield on a per sq. ft. basis because of the range of size and number of squashes per vine, from smaller and more to larger and few. All, however, like to send their vines sprawling in all directions. Some, like acorn, will creep up a fence at least a little. Be advised that acorn squash doesn't keep as well as butternut and some others.

Dry beans

By dry beans (sometimes called shell beans) I mean those that dry in the pod and have to be shelled, as opposed to green beans or snow peas, where you eat the pod as well. Dry beans are an outstanding source of protein, two-thirds as much per pound as chicken. Among the most nutritious are black, kidney, pinto, navy, and fava. Chickpeas are also nutritious, but require more care; few seed catalogues carry them.

Dry beans are so nutritious that when combined with corn and red peppers they form the core of an entire cuisine, providing almost everything you need in calories, vitamins, and minerals. No wonder they're a staple of Meso-American and many South American cultures.

There are so many amazing kinds of beans it would take the rest of the book to do them justice. Flavor varies just as much as size, color, time to cook when dried (versus fresh), and suitability for soups, baking, frying, and boiling. Yield is highest with the pole (vining) varieties, as they spread vertically, sometimes up to 8' or more. That also makes them more convenient to pick than bush varieties, which stay close to the ground and therefore require stooping or squatting to harvest. For sheer volume, of course, you get much higher yield with green beans, pole or bush, since you eat the pod as well as the bean. However, calorie-wise per unit of weight you'd come out ahead with dried beans, because they're more calorie- and protein-dense than the fleshy pods.

Sweet potatoes

Good old sweet potatoes, the official state vegetable of my home state, North Carolina. They are another source of high-calorie, high-nutrition food, rich in fiber as well as a variety of most B and C vitamins and minerals including iron, calcium, and selenium. An added benefit is that the leaves are edible, too. No wonder they're widely grown throughout the world and are the central and ancient staple of many cultures.

Interestingly, some sources claim they're low in calories, but a cup of peeled, cubed sweet potatoes has about the same number of calories—about 110 to 120—as a cup of peeled, cubed regular potatoes. The most common varieties in the U.S. are Beauregard, jewel, and garnet, also known as red yams. Sweet

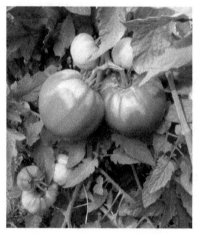

potatoes are easy to grow, and are planted not as seeds but as "slips"—rooted shoots that you either grow yourself from whole sweet potatoes or get from your local garden-goods store. Although heat- and sun-loving, they can grow just about anywhere, including Canada.

Unlike regular potatoes, you don't just pluck them out of the ground and cook them. They have to be "cured," which means storing them for a week or so at around 80° F. That causes their starch to be transformed into sugar, giving them their namesake taste. I recommend reading up on it before you try them. It's well worth your time. Which, to remind you once again, you have plenty of, to do whatever you want. Right?

Primarily for nutrients, but also with some calories

Tomatoes

Believe it or not, the most nutritious of this all-American favorite are not the red varieties but the orange ones, which most closely resemble the first cultivated tomatoes discovered in Mexico in the early 1500s. Amish Yellow Orange Oxheart, Olga's Round Golden Chicken Egg, and Orange-fleshed Purple Smudge have highest concentration of tetra-cis lycopene. It's the most nutritious form of lycopene, and the most easily absorbed by your digestive system. My favorite varieties are the pink Brandywine and almost any of the large, sweet orange varieties. One glass of high-lycopene orange tomato juice provides the same nutrition as eight glasses of red tomato juice, an advantage that is maintained even when the tomato is cooked.

However (seems like with vegetable gardening there's always a "however" or "although" lurking just around the corner), nutrition is another case where you might need to make a trade-off. The Amish Yellow Orange Oxheart, although it's denser, is a good bit smaller than pink Brandywines and other, larger, pink, orange, or red varieties. So you'd need to grow more plants to get the same output in weight. On the other hand, since they're denser, maybe you don't need to cook them down as much to get the same amount of tomato sauce. It can be fun figuring out what works best for you and gives you the most satisfaction. The possibilities are indeed endless with a garden, as any dedicated gardener will attest.

Sweet Peppers

Compared to green peppers, red bell peppers have almost 11 times as much beta-carotene, and 1.5 times as much vitamin C. Since most varieties ripen from green to red, it's simple to harvest at whatever degree of ripening suits you. Apparently no particular fully-ripened heirloom bell pepper—and they do come in a variety of colors—is more nutritious than another. But be sure to get the blocky, fleshy varieties, water them generously, and fertilize them well with compost. It's a real disappointment when you get a fairly nice-looking, good-sized pepper only to find that its walls are barely an eighth of an inch thick. Peppers are also good for drying in a dehydrator when cut into strips if they're a bell type. For the long, slender sweet varieties, just hang them in a hot, dry, sunny spot as red garlands, like they do in Italy. As with any drying process, you lose some nutrition, but judging from the centuries-old traditions of drying, there's enough left to make them a major component of many cuisines. Personally, I prefer to dice and blanch them, then store in freezer bags, making it convenient to sprinkle the pieces into a variety of soups or dishes.

Leafy Greens

Greens are easy to grow in the spring. And a second crop of some, if planted in late summer, will last well beyond freezing temperatures in the fall. The healthiest, roughly in order of nutrition, are the ever-popular kale, collards, spinach, cabbage (to be used mainly as sauerkraut), beet greens, Swiss chard, turnip greens; and lettuces such as Romaine, arugula, and endive. If you care to go to a little simple, low-tech trouble, you can insert a few heavy-wire hoops arching over your fall greens, cover them with a sheet of plastic anchored on the sides and ends with bricks, then roll it back to harvest and enjoy fresh greens down to 20°F. (Recall my somewhat fancier version thereof in Chapter 5.) Elliott Coleman takes the concept of the four-season harvest to an art form.[5] Check it out.

Carrots

Ah, the ever-famous Bugs Bunny-type orange carrots. But hold on—now, you can also get carrots that are purple, white, black, yellow, or red. Or even purple outside and orange inside. Or white inside and purple outside. Not to mention shapes and sizes that range from traditionally long and tapered, to the stubby oxheart, to a golf ball shape.

Carrots also have a fair amount of calories, but most people aren't going to eat enough carrots to put on extra weight. If they did (assuming they're gorging on traditional orange ones), the whites of their eyes would turn orange-ish from the carotenes. As happened to pilots in WWII who were fed large amounts of carrots to sharpen their eyesight, or so the story goes. Wonder what would happen if you ate gobs of purple ones . . . But those carotenes are really good for you, nonetheless.

One reviewer challenged my inclusion of carrots in the category of watery, low-calorie vegetables, probably because they're hard, like potatoes. However, you can easily make juice from carrots, but not from potatoes, beans, corn, or other high-calorie veggies. So yes, carrots are watery, just not as much so as tomatoes.

Green Beans

Although they're thought of as vegetables, green beans, also called string- or snap beans, are in the legume family along with dry beans, lentils, and peas. But they're very different from shell beans because like snow peas (another legume) the main source of nutrition is the pod, not the under-developed seeds inside. As such, they're much lower in calories than regular beans, even though they're good sources of vitamins, minerals, and fiber.

Almost everyone likes green beans. They're among the most-planted vegetables, which is why I include them here. Favorites among some hundred-plus varieties include Kentucky Wonders, Blue Lake, and Contender. They're easy to grow and prolific, whether you prefer the bush types that stay close to the ground or the climbing pole types. If you want to store them I recommend canning instead of freezing, as they tend to come out rubbery when frozen, even after cooking.

Some varieties, such as pole Kentucky Wonders, will have a more or less tough "string" (hence the name string bean) that runs the length of the pod and must be removed to make them palatable. So you can either plant one of the "stringless" types, or simply pick the beans early enough to avoid the string, as I do with pole Kentucky Wonders. A nice benefit of green beans is that if you happen to plant too many of them (easy to do) and they come on too fast to keep up with, no problem. You just let them dry in the pod and shell them as dry beans. They taste a lot like pinto beans.

Herbs

Don't forget about the herbs, starting with basil. It's easy to grow, as are oregano, dill, parsley, sage, rosemary, thyme, chives, mint, and cilantro. All, and more, will help make your garden culinary experience more savory and satisfying.

For winter, as a nutrient back-up option

Microgreens

Microgreens have become ultra-popular in recent years. You grow them from seed in dense plantings, indoors in trays, to the point where the first true foliage leaves appear. Then you cut them off at soil level and eat them fresh. They're especially good for those who crave fresh, living food in the winter when almost everything else from their garden is canned, frozen, or dried. It's also a good way to make up for the fact that when you process or store food you lose some of the nutrient content. Even a couple ounces of microgreens can be enough to fulfill the recommended daily intake of Vitamins C, E, and K. They also have a high content of anti-oxidants and minerals. By contrast, the protein, fiber, and micronutrient content is much lower per unit of weight than in regular vegetables. But then, nobody expects to subsist on microgreens alone. Rather, they're intended as a valuable nutritional supplement.

Sprouts

Sprouts were all the rage for years before microgreens appeared on the nutritional scene. They're grown from radish and other seeds, but unlike microgreens they require no substrate, and they're grown only to the point at which the cotyledons (seed leaves) appear. Then you eat the whole thing, seed and all. They also are considered to be a concentrated source of vitamins and minerals.

So which is better, microgreens or sprouts? Well, each has its benefits and drawbacks. Microgreens pack more nutrients per ounce, especially if you grow them on soil or compost rather than a sterile substrate like peat moss or coconut husk fiber. The reason is that all the nutrients in sprouts are derived from whatever is stored in the seed, whereas microgreens draw nutrients from the substrate as well as the seed. On the other hand, microgreens do require a substrate, which can't reliably be re-used due to potential soil fungus problems. Sprouts are usually grown in a jar with just water, so no substrate. But you have to be careful to rinse both the seeds and the sprouts numerous times to prevent the growth of harmful molds.

It's beyond the scope of this book to go into all the details about how to grow microgreens or sprouts, but neither is particularly difficult, and it's easy to find directions online or in books.

8

Playing the Garden
Devil's Advocate

No question, some will proclaim that a home-garden anchored food system could never make a dent in the industrial-based juggernaut, let alone largely replace it, even for just vegetables. Or that anyone other than a few gardening fanatics could actually subsist for a year on mostly or only home-grown vegetables. Never mind WWII victory gardens, examples of prodigious home-garden production in Nigeria, Cuba, and elsewhere, efficiency data from my and others' gardens, and the success of my one-month garden diet. Not to mention the Brobdingnagian lack of efficiency in our industrial system due to trillions of dollars in waste and external costs, versus negligible inefficiency for the proposed home-garden based system. Especially since it could provide much of the nation's vegetables, or even feed us entirely if need be.

Yes, I'm throwing down the gauntlet to industrial food once again. However, given the startling prospects of the humble food garden's enormous potential once implemented, I do respect the inevitable doubts. So I'll hereby play the garden devil's advocate for the benefit of all the worries, doubts, and suspicions I can think of.

Switching to mostly home gardens will cost thousands of lost jobs in the food industry

To be sure, a systemic transformation of this size and scope will bring large structural changes to agriculture- and food-related employment. But as food production begins to shift to home gardens, jobs that support and expand them will surely follow. Just as in any other sizable workforce transition, of which there have been many in the history of industrialization. For gardening, think in terms of a huge increase in the production of seeds, gardening supplies and aids, quality compost, canning and other storage supplies; gardening instruction and consultation; as well as expansion of existing and organization of new community gardens. All these areas, and more, will see a boom in new jobs that will ramp up to meet the developing demand. To serve those who get inspired by all the new home gardens but don't want to start their own, we can also expect to see a corresponding rise in the numbers of CSAs, small local farms, farmers markets, urban farms, food hubs, and the like, with concomitant employment increases.

Second, as this and other, more comprehensive books (most recently, *Food Fix* by Mark Hyman and *Perilous Bounty* by Tom Philpott, both out in 2020) have made abundantly clear, the current food system is so fundamentally flawed, abusive, and inefficient it cannot last much longer in its present form. So, drastic change is coming anyway. It absolutely has to. To give just one example, consider the fact that the automobile industry is committed to transitioning to electric vehicles within 10 to 15 years. That means that the market for 40% of the enormous U.S. corn crop devoted to ethanol will dry up, resulting in a substantial shift for the industrial supply chain of corn. Where will all that corn and attendant jobs that support it go?

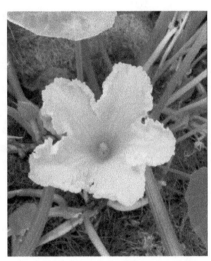

Squash Blossom

Jobs at all levels of the system—many of them extraordinarily harmful to workers—will necessarily transition to different jobs in the healthier form of food production that's coming. Hyman believes that the present food system can change and, as mentioned earlier, has prescribed over a hundred fixes he believes could make that happen. However, I really doubt that enough of those fixes could ever be implemented to render the current system sustainable. It's so deeply hidebound, misconstrued, and corrupt that trying to fix it to any significant degree would resemble the proverbial attempt to rearrange a cemetery.

Third, the switch away from predominantly industrial food production will not happen overnight, even though it will be quicker than most might anticipate. There will be time for the employment picture to shift. I think the transition to home, local, and sustainable distant systems will roll out in a timely, truly life-supporting way that will bring increased empowerment to those who need it, and relief to all of us. For the food-needy, it will be dramatically preferable to the merely stop-gap (though currently necessary) food pantries, which are by no means a permanent, healthy solution to food insecurity.

Your examples are for just one person; it's usually more complicated than that

True, but the reason I addressed growing food on a one-person basis was to keep it simple, with the idea that appropriate extrapolations could follow. The majority of people live in two- or more person households, so obviously their gardens need to be larger than mine. Of course, those homes would have more people to tend the garden, and there would likely be some economy of scale. Also, as I mentioned earlier, the required "labor" would be a benefit rather than a cost if approached the right way. Even children can help if gardening is enticingly framed as creative discovery and wonder rather than onerous weed-pulling or bean-shelling duty. In the process, they would develop a life-long delight and respect for food they'd get in no other way.

Your proposed diet is too boring to be realistic

Point well taken, since I grew only eight vegetables in my sample gardens. Based on my one-month garden diet, I know I would want more variety than that over a year, just to keep from getting totally bored. So would most other people. That's why I plan to grow a wider range of vegetables in my 2021 garden. The second and third tiers of a home-garden based system would also help fill out a more diverse diet. Still, I know from experience how empowering it is to produce for myself. As I've said before, I think that everyone should grow at least some, and ideally much of their own food. If they did, the whole country would be more food-stable, safer, and healthier, and would save a monumental amount of taxpayer money. Can't emphasize that enough.

Most people won't give up or even reduce their meat, dairy, and eggs, not to mention all the ultra-refined carbs and other goodies.

Maybe, at first. And many would never even consider having a food garden. I certainly don't plan to completely give up on all those extras myself. But I think that once people catch wind of what's going on there'll be a garden bandwagon effect. And then, watch out: it will pick up steam and riders faster than most policymakers suspect. In fact, it's already started.

Home gardeners grow mostly watery, calorie-poor vegetables, which wouldn't keep them alive for long if that were all or mostly what they ate.

I agree that you can't survive long on only watery vegetables like tomatoes, cucumbers, and zucchinis. Well, maybe you can if you eat an awful lot of them, but that would mean a much bigger garden. That is, unless you want to seriously lose weight by replacing high-calorie and ultra-processed foods with mostly low calorie vegetables while maintaining enough food volume to feel satisfied. I've never heard of such a diet, but given the never-ending parade of diet plans, it's probably out there somewhere. It could be well worth trying—with guidance from a health-food oriented dietitian or physician, of course. Maybe something like a garden vegetable version of Joe Cross's fruit and vegetable juice diet, in which he lost 82 pounds in 60 days, humorous and inspiringly documented in *Fat, Sick, and Nearly Dead.*

That's why earlier I advocated growing calorie-rich and calorie-sparse vegetables at a ratio of 2:1. If you were mining my data, you'd have noticed that for my 2020 garden vegetables, the ratio was more like 2.5:1 (228 to 92). Similarly, Table 5-6 shows that I favored calorie-rich foods by a ratio of 2.4 to 1. If home gardeners intend to subsist on their garden produce, they would likewise need to increase the proportion of calorie-rich vegetables.

Most people will never grow more than the average 15' x 20' "hobby" plot, nowhere near enough to anchor a garden-centered food system.

Even though in principle it would be relatively simple to move into home-grown as a major source of food, I realize that it could be a challenge for people to increase their current plots to something significantly larger, and to start growing more corn, beans, potatoes, winter squash, and sweet potatoes. However, the huge run in 2020 and 2021 on garden seeds, canning supplies, and even gardening accessories like tomato cages indicates that people are already more excited about gardening. The Wal-Mart in my town was even rationing canning supplies in 2020, just like toilet paper—until they ran out. And once they (and all the other stores in town that usually have canning supplies) were out, they were out for months. Those kinds of shortages went mostly under the news radar, as few national media picked up on them. So, I'd be willing to bet that we'll see evidence of even more food gardening enthusiasm come the summer of 2021. A lot more. Hopefully, suppliers will be better prepared to meet the demand.

Your claim that industrial agriculture needs three acres to feed one American for a year is hard to believe.

That figure is the average of three different estimates. The USDA reports that in 2018 there were 899.5 million acres of U.S. land in farms, including ranches.[1] Divided by our population of 331 million, that comes to 2.71 acres per person. Bloomberg says that total U.S. crop and pasture land used to produce food in 2018 was 1,007 billion acres, not counting corn and soybeans used for fuel.[2] Divide that by 331 million, and you get 3.04 acres per person. Frances Moore Lappé reported in *Diet For a Small Planet* (1982) that 3.25 acres were required to produce the Standard American Diet (SAD) per person per year.[3] In as much as U.S. agricultural exports are only 5 percent more than imports[4], trade doesn't affect the numbers appreciably. All three figures are in the same ballpark, and their average is 3.12. So for ease of discussion, I say it takes about three acres a year per American, which is very close to the Forbes estimate. Two other estimates, at 2.67[5] and 3.44[6], also average out to about 3.0.

Ironically, all these estimates are based on a "horizontal" perspective that measures only surface area, as if the amount of cropland were fixed in time. But it's not when you consider the fact that 6" is about the minimal topsoil depth required to maintain crop yields, and that it's disappearing.

A "vertical" viewpoint takes into account that, for instance in Iowa, topsoil that was about 18" deep in 1900 has been eroded to only about 6" now,[7] with most of the first 12" washed down the Mississippi to the Gulf of Mexico. That's in addition to acreage loss due to urban expansion and associated activities. Moreover, soil continues to be eroded 10 times faster than it's being replaced, even though rates of erosion have decreased in recent decades to about a third of an inch every 10 years.[8] So, we've already thrown away two entire "cake layers" of six-inch thick Iowa cropland. Each layer represents a horizontal area of some 26 million acres, or altogether 52 million, the equivalent of two agricultural Iowas, gone down the river. And we're well on our way to losing the third and final layer. Crop yields decline by 5% with each additional inch of lost topsoil.[9] That means we could expect to see a proportionate 5% increase in the area per person required to feed us for every additional inch lost.

At the rate of 1/3 inch lost every 10 years we will have lost two more inches of soil by the time today's toddlers are ready to retire 60 years from now, in 2081. That's one third of our current, remaining topsoil. With a corresponding 10% loss of yield, and thus 10% more land needed to feed us. Soil scientist Rick Cruse of Iowa State University says the real rate of topsoil loss is more like 17 times replacement[10], almost twice the above estimate. And Soil Solutions reports that at the rate at which Iowa lost topsoil between 1850 and 2000, it will be gone by 2093.[11] Unless we change the way we grow food.

Do you think switching over to scores of millions of new home food gardens while expanding the 43 million we already have might help to reverse the trend? If done properly (easy to do with mulch and compost), it would increase rather than decrease the depth of home garden topsoil, with an erosion rate of zero. It would also give millions of acres of erosion-degraded land a chance to recover.

Feeding low-income people by having them start gardens is just not credible. According to your own best figures, you'd have to have at least a 44' x 44' garden for each one of them.

Where are you going to find all that land, for free? And what if they have no interest in gardening?

Plots measuring 44'x 44'per person are not going to just pop up within existing community gardens. The first step would be to widely advertise that plots of much smaller size are available, just to get more people used to the idea that they can grow at least some of their own food. Then, as more and more get inspired and demand increases, new community gardens with increasingly larger allotments per person would be created. There has never been an effort on a national scale to create enough community garden space to address the needs of the food insecure; it would call for considerable organizational expertise and mentoring to make it all work. That's why I suggested, in Chapter 4, the figure of $25 billion to fund it. Could be it would take much less than that, maybe as little as $25 million, given the vastly lower cost of producing home-grown rather than industrial food.

There are now upwards of 66 million food-insecure Americans, and nobody really has a handle on how to enable them to start growing gardens. I don't know how to estimate the full cost of that many people going hungry, but federal expenditures for the USDA's fifteen food and nutrition assistance programs totaled $92.4 billion in 2019, with $68 billion a year for the SNAP (Supplemental Nutritional Assistance Program) alone.[12]

Making matters worse, much of the SNAP money is spent on illness-inducing junk food in response to heavy SNAP-targeted marketing. And that doesn't even take into account the cost of the many indirect social effects (e.g., diabetes in children) and economic ills (e.g., lost and inefficient work due to weakness and sickness). So yes, greatly expanded community gardens would involve significant cost, but I'd bet that, fully implemented, it would be far less than we're shelling out now for the food insecure.

As for those in need who don't find it enticing to try growing at least some of their own food, or who do but can't find or create a community garden, they will unfortunately have to continue to rely on SNAP, food pantries, or whatever other resources they can to get enough to eat. My heart goes out to them.

You aren't representative of the average American

At 5' 10.5", I weigh 140 lb., whereas the current average weight for American men is 196 lb.; for women it's 171, and for youngsters (babies to 17) it's 76. So yes, you could argue that most people weigh a good bit more than I do, and would therefore need a larger garden than mine to sustain them.

On the other hand, the prevalence of overweight and obesity in American women in 2005 was 40% for non-vegetarians vs 29% in semi-vegetarians and vegans.[13] By 2020, the rate of obesity in non-vegetarians was three times that of vegetarians.[14] The trend thus seems clear: if you're overweight—which 196 and 171 pounds are for the majority of men and women, respectively[15]— replacing at least some ultra-refined starches, sweeteners, fats, oils, dairy, and meats with vegetables is undeniably the healthy way to go. Replacing enough to reach a healthy weight (and I know that would be a daunting goal for many) would be ideal. But wouldn't it be worth the effort? Even if initially you only get part of the way toward achieving it? After all, losing 5-10% of your body weight lowers your risk of developing diabetes by 58%.[16]

In any case, since the weight of the average adult is 31% heavier than I am, increasing the size of a garden that would sustain me for a year (1,351sq. ft.) by 31% would still result in a very doable garden: 1,770 sq. ft., or 42' x 42'. That's still about 1% of the three acres industrial agriculture needs to sustain the average American.

The eight vegetables in your garden don't accurately represent the average American diet

Absolutely true. And although my garden diet would take less than 1% as much land to sustain me as the three acres the industrial system needs to feed the average American, the latter eats a *lot* of meat. More, per capita, than any other country in the world. Directly or indirectly, animal products account for over half of the land area devoted to the average diet. Another 10% is occupied by grains and other crops to produce the ultra-refined starches, sugars, oils, fats, and sweeteners we consume. To roughly compare veggies to veggies, it would theoretically take industrial food only the 5,673 square feet referred to in Chapter 4 to provide equal amounts of the kinds of (but not exactly the same) Category 1 vegetables I'd need to feed myself for a year. (See below for a more direct comparison, using the same eight vegetables I grew.) That would certainly be a more appropriate figure to cite than the three acres. Nevertheless, 5,673 square feet is still about four times as large as the 1,351 square feet it would take for me to grow the same amounts of my own vegetables.

A more direct (but much narrower) comparison would view industrial vs. my yields of the same eight vegetables I grew, using the results I obtained (for sweet potatoes, tomatoes, dry beans, kale, and snap beans) or averages for home gardens for potatoes and squash (Table 8-1). Obtained from the USDA, all of the industrial yields (cwt/acre converted to lb./sq. ft.) were recent averages for the U.S. as a whole, except for kale, for which all I could find was an average for New England.

Of the eight, sweet potatoes and tomatoes showed no significant difference; industrial yield of potatoes was about 35% higher than garden; and garden yields of squash, dry beans, snap beans, corn, and kale ranged from 5% to 210% higher than industrial. Of course, this is just eight vegetables, and only one garden, compared to millions of acres of averages for the whole country (or for kale, New England). Yet it does illustrate that a home garden can more than hold its own in vegetable yield rates compared to the industrial model.

Now, the astute reader may well ask: "You said the 5,673 sq. ft. that industrial agriculture requires to provide a year's supply of your eight vegetables per capita is about four times (400%) larger than the 1,351 square feet it would take for you to grow enough of those eight to supply yourself for a year. How can that be, given Table 8-1, which for those eight shows industrial agriculture with yield rates (except for kale) within 50% of your garden's yield rates?

Table 8-1. Garden and industrial yields of eight vegetables.
Garden is notably lower for potatoes; about the same for sweet potatoes, tomatoes, and squash; and notably higher for dry beans, kale, snap beans, and corn.

	Plot size, sq. ft.	Indust. harvest, lb.	Garden harvest, lb.	Indust. yield, lb./sq. ft.	Garden yield, lb./ sq. ft.	Garden yield, % lower or higher
Potatoes	168	168.0	124.3	1.00	0.74	-35.0
Sweet potatoes	172	68.8	67.1	0.40	0.39	-2.6
Tomatoes	161	322.0	330.1	2.0	2.05	+2.5
Squash	147	58.8	61.7	0.40	0.42	+5.0
Dry beans	168	6.7	10.1	0.04	0.06	+50.0
Kale	36	10.8	22.7	0.30	0.63	+210.0
Snap beans	126	25.2	35.3	0.20	0.28	+40.0
Corn	300	66.0	87.0	0.22	0.29	+32.0
Total		**726.3**	**738.3**			

Good question. Well, first, that 5,673 sq. ft. of industrial land is planted at one end of the food chain to cover what customers buy at the other end. Yet about half of U.S. fresh produce is wasted[17] due mostly to over-ordering, processing problems, post-harvest pest damage, and rotting along the 1,500 miles between farm and fork. Not to mention being discarded because it doesn't look pretty enough. Supermarkets alone waste some 43 billion pounds—10% of the total[18]—of perfectly good but imperfect-appearing fruits and veggies. Thus, farmers have to over-plant by 50% to make up for the 50% that's never used. So waste alone would account for half the difference between industrial yields and mine, as I can cut waste to virtually zero. For instance, when the weather got too cool for season-end tomatoes to ripen, I used every ounce of them by making 27 pints of delicious pickled green tomatoes, which I enjoy as a chunky relish every day. Even my few kitchen scraps go into the compost pile, to be applied to the next garden.

Second, there are those five vegetables for which the industry gets 5-210% less yield than I did; they would require proportionately more land than I do. But what about industrial potatoes, which get a 35% higher yield than normal for home gardens? The average American eats 116 pounds of them per year; wouldn't that largely offset higher yields for kale, snap beans, dry beans, and corn? Yes, to some degree. However, two thirds of those 116 industrial pounds are in the form of greasy, salty, nutrient-poor French fries, potato chips and "frozen or processed potato products" like tater tots.[19] Can we honestly designate such ultra-processed junk food, which technically accounts for a third of the produce that Americans consume, as vegetables in the usual sense of the word? If not, then please remove most of the yield advantage industrial potatoes have over the home-grown garden version. If you do remove them, my garden has an average 48% greater overall yield rate than the other seven industrial vegetables, which would help to account for another 25% of the yield difference. And even if you allow fries, chips, and tater tots to be counted as vegetables, my garden still averages a 38% higher yield than industrial. Just as an indication of what's possible.

A third potential reason my garden is so much more yield-efficient is the fact that my 30-day diet consisted of 2.4 parts calorie-dense to 1 part calorie-sparse vegetables. I ate a lot of corn and dry beans (Table 5-6), which are the two most calorie dense vegetables I grew. They were thus also the two most space efficient to grow in terms of area per calorie. Whereas according to the USDA, the average vegetables Americans eat—other than faux-vegetable French fries and potato chips—tend to be mostly of the low-calorie type like tomatoes and lettuce.[20] Therefore it would require much more of them, and more land per calorie to grow them, possibly accounting for the remaining 25% of the difference, than calorie-dense foods like corn and dry beans.

As an aside—and just to keep all this in perspective— we don't eat a lot of vegetables anyway. In a survey of 2,000 Americans, 25% said they never eat vegetables at all, and of the other 75%, the average person includes them in only a third of their meals.[21] Since a third of 75% amounts to an additional vegetable-free 25%, evidently around 50% of all American meals lack vegetables altogether. And that's even counting pizza—as the USDA does at the behest of Big Food lobbyists for school lunches—as a "vegetable."

Ultimately, it's probably not possible to sort out all the confounding factors when comparing the eight vegetables I grew in my garden with the same eight grown industrially on thousands of acres. Yet this much I know: relying on my well-documented rates of yield and consumption for those vegetables, I could supply myself with a year's worth of food far more efficiently—pound for pound—and considering all internal and external costs, than the industrial food system can. That is, assuming that I'd add a source of Vitamin B12, maybe a couple hens for eggs.

Which allows me to emphasize once more that I'm not saying everyone needs to be a vegetarian; I'm not one myself. But to whatever degree Americans let go of their highest-in-the-world consumption of animal protein, junk food, and sweeteners, and start growing and eating their own vegetables, the healthier they and the economy will be. And fewer will be dependent on temporary, grossly inadequate, and humiliating handouts from food pantries. How much better to eat what you are proud to have grown yourself, especially if you are food-insecure.

There's no indication among even sustainable or regenerative agriculture advocates that we should go the home garden route

It's true that none of the comprehensive plans for re-inventing the food system include a prominent, let alone leading, role for home food gardens. I think it just hasn't yet occurred to the sustainable and regenerative agriculture experts, even the most progressive ones, simply because they're so deeply locked into the idea that only farms can supply most of our food. But I've demonstrated that's simply not a valid assumption, over and over, from a number of different angles.

Furthermore—I can't stress it enough—it's the best way to quickly increase large-scale accessibility to healthy food.

Somehow your claims are just too unbelievable. Everyone knows it would take a small army of home gardeners with shovels to match what one farmer with a tractor can do.

First, recall from Chapter 2 that with standard spacing used in commercial corn production, and with the output per stalk that I achieved, home gardens would show a 35% higher yield rate, using 62% less nitrogen fertilizer, than industrial production. This is just one example of what's possible; Table 8-1 provides others.

It should not surprise anyone that a gardener's vegetable yields can easily surpass those of industrial agriculture. To begin with, garden topsoil is usually a good bit deeper than industrial soil, which as you will recall has been eroded down to about six inches and continues to be worn away at least ten times as fast as it's being replaced. That really matters, as all else being equal, yields decline 10% with the loss of each inch of soil. Moreover, industrial topsoil has lost half of its organic matter, which is important to yield because it helps to provide an easily-penetrated, loamy structure, increased fertility, and enhanced ability to hold moisture. Unlike the industrial model, most home gardens are designed to continually build up topsoil and organic matter.

The Biointensive method builds two feet of soil at one fell swoop, not a bad idea in view of the fact that the roots of most vegetables will go down at least that far in healthy soil. Home gardens can also more easily make use of succession planting, intercropping, companion planting, and winter crops, all of which increase yield. In short, the yield deck is stacked in favor of the backyard gardener.

Yes, it's at odds with the narrative that tractors and industrial production automatically out-yield gardeners with spades. But as we've seen, that isn't a forgone conclusion. Rather, what the massive use of machinery, synthetic chemicals, technology, and fossil fuels really does is enable a few people to produce food for many, which is quite different than increasing the amount of food produced per unit of land.

Most revealing, however, is not what any single component of a system can do, but what the system produces as a whole. The industrial system, of which the farmer is but one small part, produces enormous external costs in collateral health, social, economic, and environmental damage, which more than double its already huge internal costs. Beyond consideration of yield rates, those added costs drastically reduce food production efficiency overall. The contrast with home gardening, which incurs negligible external and relatively low internal costs, could hardly be greater, as both its up-front and net costs are proportionately far lower than those of industrial. The result? Compared to the industrial food system, home gardens, per pound of food currently being produced:

- Require enormously less energy
- Need much less land
- Deliver far superior health, social, economic, and environmental benefit

I challenge anyone honestly counting full costs to come up with solid evidence refuting these assertions.

Yes, but it's so much quicker and more efficient to just buy groceries in a store, or get your food from a curbside pickup or drive-through restaurant, than to grow it yourself.

On an individual basis, it certainly seems that way. But only if you ignore those monstrous external costs to the country as a whole, which you do pay for in many ways, even if you prefer not to notice it. And only if you're not one of at least 66 million Americans who don't have enough money to buy the food they need.

In other words, little-picture appearance and convenience should not be confused with big-picture efficiency and value. You lose far more than you gain when you go full-tilt industrial over home gardens, all things considered.

All that said, bear in mind that what I'm proposing is a three-tiered system that strongly favors home gardens, but is not exclusive to them.

9

Implementing a Food System Revolution

You never change things by fighting the existing reality.
To change something, build a new model that makes
the old model obsolete. —Buckminster Fuller

It's not as though no one's noticed that something is seriously wrong with the industrial food system.

Various scientists, authors, national and international institutions (including the UN), and collections of experts have been calling for a transition to something more sustainable for decades. One of the latest was the World Bank and UN-sanctioned *Agriculture at a Crossroads*, a 2018 report by the

International Assessment of Agricultural Knowledge, Science and Technology (IAASTD).[1] Reflecting input from 400 food experts from 86 countries, it proposed a multidisciplinary, multi-stakeholder plan featuring a shift from input-intensive monoculture to agro-ecology, crop diversification, small-scale farming, and local food production.

Also in 2018, the World Resources Institute's strategy promised to sustainably feed 10 billion people by 2050.[2] Even more recently, the global plan released by the Food and Land Use Coalition (FOLC) announced the *Growing Better Report 2019*,[3] which was endorsed by *Nature*, one of the most eminent scientific journals in the world. This report promised to "boost progress towards the UN's Sustainable Development Goals (SDGs) and the Paris Agreement, help mitigate the negative effects of climate change, safeguard biodiversity, ensure more healthy diets for all, drastically improve food security, and create more inclusive rural economies."

Meanwhile, the World Economic Forum's "Great Reset" proposes to transform the global food and agricultural industries to reduce food scarcity, hunger, and disease. However, it evidently favors a reductionist, high-tech approach that features GMOs, lab-made proteins, pharmaceuticals, and industrial chemicals geared more to increased corporate control over the food supply than to wholesome, healthy food.[4]

The only large-scale study about the potential of home gardens that I could find appeared in a 2013 review in the Journal *Agriculture and Food Security*.[5] It extolled the value of home gardens as a means to help address global hunger, but only for developing countries, and only as a way to supplement food from farms. This, despite instances cited in which home gardens provided 50% or more of a country's sustenance.

Regenerative organic, described briefly in Chapter 5, is getting a lot of buzz these days. Large corporations like General Mills and Cargill have pledged to regenerate millions of acres, and brands such as Nature's Path and Patagonia have received Regenerative Organic Certification. Even Wal-Mart plans to be a "regenerative" company. Yet

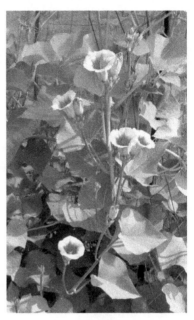

Sweet potato blossoms

regenerative still has no widely accepted definition, so how do we know who is serious about it and who's just greenwashing? Some champions of regenerative farming believe that it doesn't necessarily need to include organic concepts, so that chemical pesticides could still be used, at least at first, until they are eliminated voluntarily.

As admirable and needed as generative and other equally ambitious concepts and plans are, they will require trillions of dollars and more than a few years to significantly roll out. The FOLC reports that there are huge opportunities—valued at up to $4.5 trillion a year by 2030—for private industry to translate today's hidden food industry costs of $12 trillion per year into tomorrow's new markets. It further notes that investing in these opportunities, which will cost hundreds of billions to implement, is likely to call for "new business models that emphasize value over volume-based economics, which might require a generational shift in mindsets and leadership."

Generational? Given the world-wide pandemic and looming global recession, with ever-increasing hunger even in the U.S., do we have that kind of time right now? More to the point, are we politically prepared to invest hundreds of billions, maybe trillions, of dollars in private and/or government funds to launch a massive food-system makeover? Seems starkly unlikely, not only now but in the foreseeable future. Just to remind you of the problem's forbidding scope, Mark Hyman's comprehensive *Food Fix* proposed over a hundred industry and federal government regulatory actions needed to mitigate the corruption, waste, inequity, safety issues, and worker and consumer abuses of our food system—most of which would surely be fiercely opposed by Big Ag and Big Food. Fortunately for us, he also recommended 37 personal steps we can take to take to protect ourselves while we're waiting (for how long?) for those fixes to happen.

That's why ramping up a garden-anchored system, which we don't have to wait around for, has much greater potential for delivering reliable food. Compared to what it would take to even think about changing the vast industrial system, expanding home gardening is refreshingly easy for the average person to grasp and embrace. Gardens promise to act as a powerful lever for addressing the failures of our present system not only because of their simplicity, but also because they turn on the fulcrum of being simultaneously voluntary, efficient, effective, and enjoyable.

Home gardens are also better positioned than local food systems to quickly increase food production and accessibility on a national scale. In 2015, CSAs accounted for only 0.02%[6] of U.S. grocery sales of some $683 billion,[7] and their prices are still undercut by industrial food trucked in from thousands of miles away. Similarly, sales direct from farms to consumers come in at only $3 billion annually,[8] about 0.4% of total grocery sales. Even the "booming" farmers markets, though steadily increasing, still constitute only a tiny fraction of the overall food market.

By contrast, it bears repeating that over a third of all U.S. households already have a home food garden, and 67% of adults say they have a food garden or are thinking of starting one.[9] The point is, the infrastructure for home food gardens is already largely in place, far more widely developed, and with much greater immediate potential to ramp up. That is, compared to CSAs, farmers markets, and the like. In effect, home gardens are primed, ready and able to pounce. Yet when they do, I predict that they will not compete with, but rather, will provide a welcome boost to the CSAs and their kin.

Home and community gardens also have the aforementioned perks that local food systems can't fully match, such as reconnecting people to nature while providing enjoyable exercise and self-empowered food security. Labor, counted as a cost (and it's huge) in industrial as well as local agriculture, becomes a benefit when employed at a voluntary and healthy scale in home gardens.

Again, I'm not suggesting that we get rid of industrial food altogether, much less abandon the local food system, which we do need. Rather, that home gardens be the anchor, complemented by the local scene, which in turn could be complemented by an industrial system that has evolved, hopefully at a scale that's reduced enough to correct its unsustainable features.

In short, a system anchored by home food gardens can feed us cheaper, faster, healthier, and much better than pure industrial. Let's take a look at the broad outlines of what it would take to make that happen.

Guiding concepts for gardeners

For the current food gardener

You already know what to do; just do more of it. That is, expand your garden and start thinking in terms of meaningful production to see how long you could sustain yourself. Doesn't have to be for a whole year, just start heading in that direction to see what you can accomplish enjoyably.

For the aspiring new gardener

Start up a food garden, no matter how small at first; the point is not how large it is to begin with, but just to begin.

For both:

It absolutely must be voluntary, including for kids. Don't force them to garden; rather, entice and charm them by genuine, enthusiastic example, with the intention of allowing the plants themselves to be the primary charmers.

- It has to be enjoyable, because only to the degree that it's fun and inspiring will it be worthwhile. If it's not, but you still want to do it, or you make an initial effort that doesn't go anywhere, don't let yourself to be overcome by garden guilt. Step back a little and consider what will make it truly enjoyable and more lasting. Do you find it too difficult, physically too demanding? Then either change your tactics (with more help from gardening resources, friends, or gardening mentors) or put up a notice on your neighborhood bulletin board announcing that you would like some assistance. If you don't get any volunteer takers, don't be shy about offering a little pay for a teenager or even younger helper; they would love it. Or get your local Boy and/ or Girl Scouts involved. Or church groups, or gardening clubs. Whatever it takes.

- Although just getting started is most important, at some point you may want to favor those calorie-rich veggies about 2:1 over the calorie-sparse ones. That will best serve you if your longer-term goal is to see how much of your own food you can grow, and how long you can make it last.

- Devise a way to assess how long your garden could support you if you had to depend on it for all your food, based on the your rates of yield and consumption of what you grow, and assuming a 2:1 ratio of calorie-rich to low calorie vegetables. Then use that to plan your gardens, gradually ramping up your self-sufficiency quotient (total self-sufficient days divided by 365) according to what you find enjoyable to produce and satisfying to eat.

- At some point, do your own Garden Super-Size Me experiment. Could you eat only from your garden for just one meal? For a day? A whole week? If you do, what's it like? How does it make you feel? You won't know until you try it. So, try it. I think you'll be amazed at how fulfilling it is, and how it will inspire you.

Guiding concepts and steps for policymakers

Step up and decide it's time to unequivocally address food sustainability

The decades of dithering are over. It really is time to act. The pandemic crisis should galvanize us to boldly reach out and do things in the "New Truth" (post-COVID-19 arrival) that we wouldn't have seriously considered in the "Before Times" (pre-COVID). Then, once we decide to act, we need to implement the most effective strategies to largely re-invent food production as quickly and effectively as possible.

Fortunately, we don't need to start from scratch, either practically or conceptually. We simply need to expand upon the example set by those who are already doing the right thing: home gardeners. To give credit where it's due, theirs are the sturdy shoulders we should be grateful to stand on.

Make home gardens the anchor of the food system, backed by local food sources, complemented by more distant food sources

The proportion of food produced in each of these levels will be flexible, but will shift overall from the current heavy emphasis on the industrial end to the local and home food end. The pace of the shift, the degree to which food produced in the industrial tier moves to the other tiers, and the way the whole transformation will play out in different geographical regions, will vary.

Internalize all costs at all three tiers of the new food system

If there is any one, unifying, powerful lever that encapsulates the entire proposition of this book, this would be it. The current system doesn't know how to, cannot, and will not internalize its costs. It doesn't even want to. I would even go so far as to stay that the only way that all costs of food production can be internally accounted for is to move to the proposed three-tiered system. Local food systems will greatly help, but alone won't be enough to get rid of the industry's concept that it's okay to foist more than half of your costs off onto others.

Simply put, internalization, or full-cost accounting, means that all participants at all tiers pay their costs either immediately or in a timely manner. That doesn't prohibit temporary subsidies or incentives to effect the transition to new practices, but it does mean repaying those and other forms of loans reasonably quickly. That is, not becoming dependent on them indefinitely, as has been the case for decades with "farmer welfare" in the industrial system. Through which, not incidentally, it's not farmers but corporate middlemen who indirectly end up with the lion's share of those welfare checks.

Not moving to internalizing costs is what has made it structurally impossible for the industrial system to effectively cope with COVID-19, especially for the food insecure.

Prioritize those most in need

Although the national media is documenting change, it's astonishing how it still focuses more on revised shopping habits of those who still have enough money to buy food than on those who have to "shop" at food pantries. It's high time to put the latter first, not last, in creating new food strategy responses. Again, *first*, not *last*. This is key not only with respect to the pandemic but also with regard to the underlying, pre-COVID condition of food insecurity.

Make initiatives voluntary, but provide extensive support

No matter who is coordinating or helping to foment it, gardening should be not only voluntary and from the ground up as much as possible. That is, no mandates, no command and control attitudes or strategies should be invoked to force people to garden; that would only generate resentment and push-back. Encouragement, example, and inspiration, already the spirit of effective gardening help, should be the spirit of a home-gardening campaign.

Assemble and coordinate multi-level teams to promote home gardens

The USDA did an amazing job of promoting, guiding, and helping people to set up the WWII victory gardens, and now it has a People's Garden website that provides tools and resources for gardeners to start or expand a home, school, or community garden. In addition, it has an infrastructure already in place to implement it: the County Extension Offices present in every state. It would be highly desirable for the Extension Service to help set up a network of home gardening organizers and mentors in every community.

Ahead of the game is the National Gardening Association, which has been promoting gardening, including food gardens, since 1971. It offers a gardening primer to help newbies get started. For those who don't have their own land, or suitable land to start a garden, the American Community Gardening Association could step up to assist.

In addition to those resources are many other private initiatives and associations, including the Home Garden Association, the Master Gardener Association, and any number of in-person and online vegetable planning courses and websites. These efforts to spread vegetable gardening should extend not only to personal yards but also to schools, from pre-Kindergarten to college, and to hospitals and businesses that have open sunny spaces. Likewise, efforts should be made to foster the expansion of all the support services that will be needed to meet a boom in home food gardening. That begins with affordable, high-quality compost and well-informed instruction in gardening methods.

It's especially important that all of these services be made accessible to those who have no space to garden, and few or no resources. A national network of organizers should be established to foster the creation of new community gardens where they're needed but don't exist. And all of them should be designed to serve everyone, including homeless people, for free if that's what it takes to entice them into participating,.

Inspiration at the top will greatly help. That means re-invigorating the vegetable garden that Michelle Obama so audaciously started on the White House lawn; it was graciously continued, though less enthusiastically, under Melania Trump. However, it has been maintained by the National Park Service with a $1.2 million budget. While Michelle's garden is commendable for its symbolism, inspiration, and beauty, I suggest that a second garden be dedicated to meeting the food needs of an average, healthy person for a year on a household budget, maintained by an average gardener. Maybe it could be at another location within the White House grounds, so as not to be seen as competing with the existing garden. In this way, a garden the size of mine, maybe a little larger, could serve as an attainable example. If a 72-year old can be largely food self-sufficient with a few hand tools, simple fences, and a wheelbarrow, "working" an average of at most 30 minutes a day, most others could also. Call it regenerative rather than organic, because that word is both more meaningful and less off-putting than organic, at least to some people. Going beyond outward appearances, at least some of the vegetables it produces should appear regularly in the presidential cuisine (as evidently those of Michelle's garden did), and even in formal state dinners, with the press prominently heralding every such event.

Likewise, there should be model regenerative gardens on the lawns of state capitols and town squares, rendering the concept even more visible. One nice thing about growing your own vegetables is it's free of politics and other potentially divisive arenas. Democrat or Republican, conservative or progressive, Christian, Muslim, atheist, or whatever, growing a vegetable garden can be included among the values of people of any persuasion; that's how fundamental the principles of wholesome food and self-sufficiency are. We all have to eat, and we all like to be able to take care of ourselves.

Celebrities could also contribute enormously, not only financially (especially to community garden organization) but more importantly, by example. I recently saw where LeBron James, who many consider to be the world's number one basketball player, decided to switch from endorsing Coca Cola to Pepsi. Much as I respect and admire him, I winced. Sugary soft drinks are a major contributor to the obesity epidemic. How much better it would have been to switch to endorsing juices made from organic fresh vegetables. Especially since millions of kids look up to him. Likewise, thought leaders and celebrities from not only sports but also entertainment, religion, business, education, the arts, politics, and of course the world of food, could lead by example. Busy as they are, if they could show that they have a vegetable plot that they personally tend to regularly, even if it's only once a week (hiring someone to watch it when they can't be there), it would set a powerfully inspiring example.

Wait, LeBron James tending a garden? Is that even remotely realistic? (I can just imagine Charles Barkley letting out a huge laugh.) Well, there *is* the off season. And remember, just like you and me, LeBron and other, equally busy celebrities (I'm looking at you, too, Charles) always have the time to do what they want to do. Right?

As for the future, here's my ultimate milestone of acceptance: when we start seeing demonstration food gardens on the spacious decks of those big ocean liners, with freshly harvested items proudly identified in their restaurant menus and incorporated into at least some of the meals they serve, we will know that food gardens tended directly and lovingly by human hands have achieved their rightful status.

The bigger picture

Overall, the proposed transition to a home-garden anchored food system isn't just about delivering access to quality food. More fundamentally, it's about delivering permanent relief from current food problems by creating new value. All genuine economic value is created in the same basic way that plants use the air to create food and oxygen with the help of sunlight and a tiny bit of nutrients from the ground. That is, by transforming something of less worth into something of greater—and genuine—value. By genuine I mean value that extends to all, not just to some at the expense of others. As we transition to the "New Truth" we will increasingly need to find new ways to create new value in all areas of life as a foundation for new production systems serving a truly healthy society. Food gardens can lead the way by showing us how.

Most important for making all this happen will be generating a widespread, informed attitude, so that gardeners everywhere, as well as various government and private organizations, will be inspired to cooperate. For the food insecure it will bring long-term dignity, pride, and self-sufficiency in a way that food pantries never could. Although getting enough quality calories and nutrients is the practical goal, real, permanent food security is about so much more, for everyone. Ultimately, it means restoring our flexibility, power, and well-being as we re-connect ourselves with one of the most enjoyable impulses of what it means to be human: creating and consuming healthy food.

Appendix 1

Yield and cost performance of heirloom red grits and cornmeal compared to commercial grits and cornmeal

Basic data

- There are 56 lb. of corn in a bushel
- There are 43,560 sq. ft. in an acre
- A 15' x20' plot = 300 sq. ft.
- Standard spacing for maximum yield of corn is 30" between rows, 6" between plants in a row
- In 2019 the U.S. commercial yield of corn averaged 168 bu./acre

My yield in 2019

- My 2019 corn plot consisted of 4 rows, 4' apart and 22' long
- There were 25 plants per row with an average spacing of 0.875' (= 10.5") between plants, for a total of 100 plants
- Area of the plot: 4 x (4' x 22')= 352 sq. ft.
- From that plot I harvested 36 lb. shelled, well-dried corn
- 100 plants/36 lb.= 0.36 lb. of corn per plant

Potential for maximum yield

- To maximize yield, I would need to increase plants per row and the number of rows:
- In a 15' x 20' plot, I would plant six 20' rows 30" apart, and 6" between plants in a row (15' x 12"/ft= 180" per row; 180"/30" per row = 6 rows; 6" spacing = 0.5')
- 20'/row x 2 plants/ft = 40 plants/row
- 40 plants/row x 6 rows = 240 plants
- 240 plants x 0.36 lb./plant = 86.4 lb. of corn from a 300 sq. ft. plot
- 86.4 lb./300 sq. ft. = 0.29 lb./sq. ft.
- 43,560 sq. ft./acre x 0.29 lb./sq. ft. = 12,632 lb./acre
- 12,632 lb./acre/56 lb./bu. = 226 bu. /acre
- = 26% higher rate of yield than the 2019 U.S. average corn yield, which = 168 bu./acre

Profit from my 2019 corn plot

- Size of plot: 16' x 22'
- 36 lb. of harvested, dried corn
- My processed ratio of dried corn to grits and cornmeal is 2:1, or 0.67 to 0.33
- So, from 36 lb. of corn I would get:
  o 36 lb. x 0.67 = 24 lb. of grits; 36 lb. x 0.33 = 12 lb. of cornmeal
  o Market price of my grits = $13.97/lb.
  o Market price of my cornmeal =$9.92/lb.

- o $13.97/lb. x 24 lb. = $335.28 for grits
- o $9.92/lb. x 12 lb. = $119.04 for corn
- o Total value $454.32
- o Return on investment = $454 for $4 worth of seed and a few tablespoons of organic liquid fertilizer (not counting fixed costs of a gardening spade and protective fencing, which have been used for many years)

Potential profit I would get from a 15' x 20' plot with standard spacing for corn

- 86.4 lb. of corn from a 15' x 20' plot (= 300 sq. ft.)
- My processed ratio of dried corn to grits and cornmeal is 2:1, or 0.67 to 0.33
- So, from 86.4 lb. of corn I would get:
  - o 86.4 lb. x 0.67 = 57.9 lb. of grits; 86.7 lb. x 0.33 = 28.5 lb. of cornmeal
  - o The market price of my grits is $13.97/lb.
  - o The market price of my cornmeal is $9.92/lb.
  - o $13.97/lb. x 57.9 lb. = $808.86 for grits
  - o $9.92/lb. x 26.4/lb. = $261.89 for corn
  - o Total value $1,070.75
  - o Return on investment = $1,071 for $8 of seed (not counting fixed costs of gardening spade and protective fencing, which have been used for many years)

Conclusion: at least for a 15' x 20' plot of corn planted at standard spacing, which anyone could do in their back yard, given enough sun and gardening know-how, it's simply not true that yield rates of industrial agriculture outperform those of small scale farming. This is powerful knowledge.

Proportion of U.S. corn consumed directly by Americans that backyard gardens could provide

- There are about 128 million households in the U.S.
- Approximately 80% of all households in the U.S. have lawns
- Therefore 128 x 0.8 = 102 million homes have lawns
- The average size of the American yard is 10,871 sq. ft., so we can assume most lawns will have 300 sq. ft.
- 300 sq. ft. of lawn area can produce 86.4 lb. of corn using standard spacing for corn plants
- 1 bu. of corn weighs 56 lb.
- So 86.4 lb./lawn/56 lb./bu. = 1.54 bu./lawn
- 102 million lawns x 1.54 bu./lawn = 144 million bu.

U.S. corn yield in 2018-19 was 14.42 billion bu.

However, less than 10% of the corn used in the United States is directly ingested by humans, and much of that is used for high-fructose corn syrup.[1]

If 10% of the U.S. corn crop was directly ingested by humans, that would be:

- 0.1 x 14.42 billion bu. = 1.44 billion bu.
- 1.44 million bu./1.42 billion bu. = 0.10 = 10%

So if every home that had a yard grew a 15' x 20' plot of corn with standard plant spacing, and got the same amount of corn per plant that I did, it would more than cover the proportion of the U.S. corn crop currently devoted to direct human consumption.

The other 90% of the U.S. corn crop, used for processed human food, animal feedstock, fuel, and industrial purposes, would still have to be produced by conventional farming.

Appendix 2

Nitrogen Fertilization of my Corn vs. Commercial U.S. Corn

Nitrogen in human urine

"Our urine contains significant levels of nitrogen, as well as phosphorous and potassium. The relative ratios are typically around 11 parts nitrogen to 1 part phosphorus to 2.5 parts potassium. Americans produce about 90 million gallons of urine a day, containing about seven million pounds of nitrogen."[1]

Nitrogen, by weight, in lb., in a cup of urine

- 7 m lb. of N/90 m gal. of urine = 0.08 lb. of N/gal. of urine
- There are 16 cups in a gallon, so:
  - (0.08 lb./gal) / (16 cups/gal) = 0.005 lb. of N/cup of urine

Fertilization dilution rate

- Pour 3 cups of urine into a 2-gallon watering can, then fill it with water
- There are 32 cups in 2 gallons

- 3 cups urine/32 cups of urine-diluted water = 0.09 cups urine/cup of urine-diluted water. (Hereafter I refer to urine-diluted as "N-diluted")

Nitrogen, by weight, applied to each corn plant

- I used 1 cup of N-diluted water to fertilize each plant per application
- 0.09 cup urine/cup N-diluted water x 0.005 lb. of N/cup urine
- = 0.0004 lb. N/application/plant

My corn

- I applied six cups of N-diluted water to each plant (1 cup every 2 weeks over 12 weeks)
- 0.0004 lb. N/application/plant x 6 applications /plant = 0.0024 lb. N/plant (total)
- Consider six 20' rows 2.5' between rows: (6 rows) x (20'/row) x (2.5') = 300 sq. ft.
- I planted 2 plants/ft. within a row, so 2 plants/ft. x 20' row = 40 plants/row
- 40 plants/row x 6 rows = 240 plants in a 300 sq. ft. plot
- 0.0024 lb. N/plant x 240 plants/300 sq. ft./plot = 0.576 lb. N/ 300 sq. ft./plot
- There are 43,560 sq. ft. in an acre
- 43,560 sq. ft./acre/300 sq. ft./plot = 145, 300 sq. ft plots/acre
- 145 plots/acre x 0.576 lb./plot = 83 lb. N/acre

According to *Emergence by FBN*, "Corn plants use large quantities of nitrogen to grow and yield. Corn removes 1 pound of nitrogen for every bushel of grain produced, so a 250 bushel per acre yield goal requires 250 pounds of nitrogen available to be used by your growing corn plants."[2]

Yet with an application rate of 83 lb. N/acre I got a yield rate of 226 bu./acre

So, my N application rate was 83 lb. N/acre/226 bu./acre =0.37 lb. N/bu.

- Penn State University Extension says to apply 220 lb. N/acre to get an expected yield of 200 bu./acre[3]
- 220 lb. N/acre/200 bu./acre/ = 1.1 lb. N/bu., about what *Emergence* stated
- Comparing my N usage rate to Penn State's expected N use rate, i.e., the ratio of my rate to their recommended use rate:
  o 0.37 lb. N/bu./1.1 lb. N/bu. = 0.34
  o So, I got a 34% higher rate of yield (226 bu./acre) than the 2019 U.S. corn yield (168 bu./acre) applying only 34% of the N/acre recommended to get a yield of 200 bu./acre.
  o This compellingly contradicts the industry narrative that conventional agriculture is far more efficient than backyard gardening.

Here's a secondary check, from another angle

According to an article in *Scientific American* on the U.S. corn system, over 5.6 million tons of nitrogen are used on U.S. corn each year.[4] Using that figure, along with the 2019 corn yield of 14.42 billion bu., one can determine the lb. of N used per bu. of corn:

- So, 5,600,000 tons of N x 2,000 lb./ton = (5.6 x 10^6 tons of N) x (2.0 x 10^3 lb./ton) = 11.2 x 10^9 lb. of N
- U.S. corn yield in 2018-19 was 14.42 billion bu,= 14.42 x 10^9 bu
- (11.2 x 10^9 lb. of N) / (14.42 x 10^9 bu) = 0.78 lb. N/bu.
- 0.78 lb. N/bu = 1/0.78 lb.N/bu = 1.3 bu/lb. N

The main form of N in human urine is urea, which also accounts for 70% of all industrial N used as fertilizer, so it's reasonable to compare the weight of nitrogenous compounds of my fertilizer with that in the commercial form.

Coming back to the claim that each bushel of corn requires a pound of N used, I got 2.7 bu. of corn per pound of N applied. It's not likely that there was an additional 1.7 lb. of N per bu. already in the soil. Besides, soil bacteria process a lot of applied N, only a fraction of which is made available for corn uptake, and probably some N in the liquid fertilizer I used leached through to the subsoil. So according to this reckoning, my gardening methods evidently utilize N at least two times as efficiently as commercial corn production methods while producing a 34% higher rate of yield.

Further discrediting the claim of industrial scale efficiency, it takes huge amounts of energy to produce the needed N fertilizer per bushel of commercial corn compared to zero energy to produce the N fertilizer needed per bushel of my corn.

Says David Pimental of Syracuse, "It takes 800 liters of oil (5 barrels of oil) per ha. of corn produced in the USA. A third of this energy goes to making N fertilizer, another third for machinery and fuel, and the final third goes to herbicides, irrigation, and other fertilizers."[5]

For the squeamish, diluting 1 part urine to 9 parts water:

- Urine is 5% solids and 95% water
- Which is 1 part solids to 19 parts water = $1/20^{th}$ solids
- The dilution I used is 1 part urine to 9 parts water
- So, solids in the fertilizer solution = $1/10^{th}$ of $1/20^{th}$
- = 1 part solids in 2,000 parts water
- Not only that, the solids, including those that contain nitrogen, are tasty to soil microbes that gobble them up and process them into forms that can then be taken up by plant roots

Does that make it a little easier?

Of course, you could always just use compost, perfectly fine and the usual way to responsibly fertilize anyway, although it's fairly low in nitrogen if it's mature. But the grand irony would be people being squeamish about using human urine on a very small, clean scale when industrial CAFOs collect pools of thousands of tons of liquid livestock waste that stinks up the countryside for miles around, is often then spread fresh on agricultural fields, and pollutes ground and surface waters.

Notes

Chapter 1

1   Dobberstein, J. "Do We Still Have Only 60 Harvests
    Left?" No-Till Farmer, March 25, 2020. https://www.
    no-tillfarmer.com/blogs/1-covering-no-till/post/9569-
    do-we-still-only-have-60-harvests-left.

2   Hyman, M. *Food Fix – How to Save Our Health, Our
    Economy, Our Communities, and Our Planet – One Bite at a
    Time.* Little, Brown, Spark. 2020.

Chapter 2

1   Wunsch, Nils-Gerrit. "Per Capita Consumption of Corn
    Products in the U.S. from 2000-2019." Statista. Nov
    26, 2019. https://www.statista.com/statistics/184202/
    per-capita-consumption-of-corn-products-in-the-us-
    since-2000/

2   "The Declining Nutrient Value of Food." Mother
    Earth News. Editorial. December 2011 / January 2012.
    https://www.motherearthnews.com/homesteading-and-
    livestock/nutrient-value-of-food-zm0z11zphe

3   "Growing Louisville: The benefits of urban and
    community gardening." Louisville. May 22, 2015.
    https://archive.louisville.com/content/growing-
    louisville-benefits-urban-and-community-gardening.

4   Langellotto, G.A, "What are the Economic Costs
    and Benefits of Home Vegetable Gardens?" *Journal of
    Extension*, April, 2014. 52:2rb5.

5   Rouse, L. "The Surprising Economics of Vegetable
    Gardening," Wrkf89.3. May 6, 2017. https://www.wrkf.
    org/post/surprising-economics-vetegable-gardening.

6 Perry, L. "Why Grow Vegetables?" University of Vermont Extension, Winter/Spring. https://pss.uvm.edu/ppp/articles/whygrow.html

7 Dobsevage, R. "What's a Garden Worth? Roger and Jacqueline Doiron Do the Math and Calculate the Cost of Their Garden Vegetables for One Growing Season." https://www.finegardening.com/article/whats-a-garden-worth

8 Blume, D. Food and Permaculture. http://www.permaculture.com

9 Jeavons, J. Interview: Biointensive Method Continues to Help Farmers Reap Ultra-Productive Harvests, Boost Soil Health. Eco-Farming Daily. https://www.ecofarmingdaily.com/biointensive-method-continues-help-farmers-reap-ultra-productive-harvests-boost-soil-health/

10 Ambrose, G., Das, K., Fan, Y., and Ramaswami, A. "Is gardening associated with happiness of urban residents? A mult-activity, dynamic assessment in the Twin-Cities region, USA." Landscape and Urban Planning, June, 2020. https://www.sciencedirect.com/science/article/pii/S0169204619307297?via%3Dihub

11 Garden to Table. National Gardening Association. A 5-Year Look at Food Gardening in America. 2014.

12 Cunningham, W.P. and Cunningham, M.A. *Environmental Science – A Global Concern.* 2018.

Chapter 3

1   Corkery, M. and Yaffe-Bellany. "We Had to Do Something: Trying to Prevent Massive Food Waste." May 2, 2020. *The New York Times*. https://www.nytimes.com/2020/05/02/business/coronavirus-food-waste-destroyed.html

2   Yashking. "Why Food Banks are So Overwhelmed Right Now," MNN. Newsfragment. May 18, 2020. https://newsfragment.com/why-food-banks-are-so-overwhelmed-right-now-mnn/

3   Abel, David. "I've Never Seen Anything Like This Kind of Need: Food Pantries Struggle to Keep Up with Surge in Demand." Nov. 24, 2020. *The Boston Globe*. https://www.treehugger.com/food-banks-struggling-coronavirus-pandemic-4859439#:~:text=According%20to%20Feeding%20America%2C%2059,afraid%20they'll%20need%20them.

4   Lowery, A. "The Second Great Depression – At Least Four Major Factors are Terrifying Economists and Weighing on the Recovery." June 23, 2020. The Atlantic. https://www.theatlantic.com/ideas/archive/2020/06/second-great-depression/613360/

5   Hazimihalis, K. "These Grocery Store Waste Statistics are a Wake-Up Call." Oct. 31, 2018. Dumpsters.com Blog. https://www.dumpsters.com/blog/grocery-store-food-waste-statistics

6   Kornfield, M. "COVID-19 Has Killed 100 Grocery Store
     Workers. Vitalina Williams Was One of the First." *The
     Washington Post*. May 27, 2020. https://www.boston.com/
     news/coronavirus/2020/05/27/covid-19-has-killed-100-
     grocery-store-workers-vitalina-williams-was-one-of-the-
     first/

7   USDA Economic Research Service. "Food Security
     and Nutrition Assistance." Dec 16, 2020. https://www.
     ers.usda.gov/data-products/ag-and-food-statistics-
     charting-the-essentials/food-security-and-nutrition-
     assistance/#:~:text=In%202019%2C%2089.5%20
     percent%20of,than%202018%20(11.1%20percent)

8   "The Impact of the Coronavirus on Food Insecurity."
     Feeding America. April 22, 2020. https://www.
     feedingamerica.org/sites/default/files/2020-04/
     Brief_Impact%20of%20Covid%20on%20Food%20
     Insecurity%204.22%20%28002%29.pdf

9   Food Insecurity. Northwestern Institute for Policy
     Research. July 2020. https://www.ipr.northwestern.edu/
     what-we-study/trending-policy-topics/food-insecurity.
     html

10   Guest. "Startling Drone Footage Shows 1.5 Mile-Long
     Line of Cars Waiting Outside a Drive-Thru Food Bank
     in Miami that Gives Out 2.5 million Meals Per Week
     as Coronavirus Effects Leave Millions Hungry." March
     15, 2020. https://feedingsouthflorida.org/1-5-mile-long-
     line-of-cars-waits-outside-a-drive-thru-food-bank-for-
     food-distribution/

11 Fowler, G. "In 2020, We Reached Peak Internet. Here's
    What Worked – and What Flopped." Dec. 28, 2020. *The
    Washington Post*. https://www.washingtonpost.com/
    topics/road-to-recovery/2020/12/28/covid-19-tech/

12 Community Gardens in New Orleans. Wikipedia.
    https://en.wikipedia.org/wiki/Community_gardens_in_
    New_Orleans

13 Research Regarding the Benefits of
    Community Gardens. N.C. State Extension.
    https://nccommunitygardens.ces.ncsu.edu/
    nccommunitygardens-research/

14 Grabell, M., Pearlman, C., and Yeung, B. "Emails reveal
    chaos as meatpacking companies fought health agencies
    over COVID-19 outbreaks in their plants." June 12,
    2020. *Propublica*. https://www.propublica.org/article/
    emails-reveal-chaos-as-meatpacking-companies-fought-
    health-agencies-over-covid-19-outbreaks-in-their-plants

15 Kindy, K. "More than 200 meat plant workers in the U.S.
    have died of COVID-19. Federal regulators just issued
    two modest fines." Sept 13, 2020. *The Washington Post*.
    https://www.washingtonpost.com/national/osha-covid-
    meat-plant-fines/2020/09/13/1dca3e14-f395-11ea-
    bc45-e5d48ab44b9f_story.html

16 Meyer, Jane. "How Trump is helping tycoons exploit the
    pandemic." July 20, 2020. https://www.newyorker.com/
    magazine/2020/07/20/how-trump-is-helping-tycoons-
    exploit-the-pandemic

17 Ibid.

18 Robinson, M. Jorge's Organics: "A flourishing family
    greenhouse." Apr. 6, 2020. The Iowa Source. https://www.
    iowasource.com/2020/04/06/jorges-organics/

19 Changes in USDA food composition data for 43 garden
    crops, 1950 to 1999." Journal of the American College
    of Nutrition. 23: 669-82. December 2004. https://www.
    researchgate.net/publication/8094536_Changes_in_
    USDA_Food_Composition_Data_for_43_Garden_
    Crops_1950_to_1999#:~:text=A%20comparison%20
    of%20nutritional%20quality,et%20al.%2C%202004)%20.

20 Have Fruits and Vegetables Become Less Nutritious?"
    March 17, 2020. Global Heart. https://globalheart.nl/
    gezondheid/have-fruits-and-vegetables-become-less-
    nutritious/

21 Ibid.

22 Ibid.

23 "Vegetables lose half of their nutritional value by the
    time they get to the store: Another reason to grow your
    own." Return to Now. Sept. 23, 2018. https://returntonow.
    net/2018/09/23/study-produce-loses-around-half-its-
    vitamin-content-within-a-week-of-harvest/

24 Karthikeyan, V. and Garber, A. "How safe is our food?
    Recent trends and case studies of recalls, and what they
    mean for our health." U.S. PIRG. https://uspirg.org/
    feature/usp/how-safe-our-food#:~:text=Americans%20
    should%20be%20confident%20that,coli%20and%20
    Salmonella.&text=The%20Centers%20for%20
    Disease%20Control,and%203%2C000%20dying%20
    every%20year.

25 Ducharme, J. "You're not imagining it: Food recalls are
    getting more common. Here's why." Jan. 17, 2019. Time.
    https://time.com/5504355/food-recalls-more-common/

26 "A look back at 2019 Food Recalls." March 17, 2020. *Food Safety Magazine*. https://www.foodsafetymagazine.com/ enewsletter/a-look-back-at-2019-food-recalls/

27 Ducharme, J. "You're not imagining it: Food recalls are getting more common. Here's why." Jan. 17, 2019. *Time*. https://time.com/5504355/food-recalls-more-common/

28 Ibid.

29 Calderone, J. "How safe is your kids' food? A new report highlights food additives that may be harmful to kids. Here are 5 steps to take to keep kids safer." July 24, 2018. *Consumer Reports*.

30 Twilley, N. "When a virus is the cure." Dec. 21, 2020. *The New Yorker*. https://www.newyorker.com/ magazine/2020/12/21/when-a-virus-is-the-cure

31 "Human Health – Toxic emissions from industrial farms are having serious adverse health effects on U.S. citizens." https://agreenerworld.org/challenges-and-opportunities/ human-health/?gclid=EAIaIQobChMIoPbg2ev16gIVk 8DACh3yYgsIEAAYAyAAEgJprPD_BwE

32 Roseboro, K. "The coming obsolescence of GMO seeds." The organic and non-GMO report. February 8, 2021. https://non-gmoreport.com/articles/the-coming-obsolescence-of-gmo-seeds/

33 Lawrence, F. "Rotten meat and bottled formaldehyde: fighting for food safety." Oct. 15, 2018. *Nature*. https:// www.nature.com/articles/d41586-018-07038-0

34 Bhattarai, A. and Denham, H. "Stealing to survive: More Americans are shoplifting food as aid runs out during the pandemic." Dec.10, 2020. *The Washington Post.* https://www.washingtonpost. com/business/2020/12/10/pandemic-shoplifting-hunger/?utm_campaign=wp_post_most&utm_medium=email&utm_source=newsletter&wpisrc=nl_most&carta-url=https%3A%2F%2Fs2.washingtonpost. com%2Fcar-ln-tr%2F2d727db%2F5fd24e939d2fda0efb 8453ca%2F5978b1faae7e8a6816eb45fd%2F8%2F66%2F 5fd24e939d2fda0efb8453ca

35 Hyman, M. *Food Fix – How to save our health, our economy, our communities, and our planet – one bite at a time.* Little, Brown, Spark. 2020.

36 Popkin, G. "Is carbon sequestration on farms actually working to fight climate change?" *GreenBiz.* Apr. 16, 2020. https://www.greenbiz.com/article/carbon-sequestration-farms-actually-working-fight-climate-change

37 Coffey, D. "Could we ever pull enough carbon out of the atmosphere to stop climate change?" Space.com. https://www.space.com/can-carbon-removal-slow-climate-change.html

38 Regenerative organic agriculture and climate change. A down to earth solution to climate change. Rodale Institute. https://rodaleinstitute.org/wp-content/uploads/Regenerative-Organic-Agriculture-White-Paper. pdf

Chapter 4

1 "Total retail and food sales in the United States from 1992 to 2019." *Statista.* July 24, 2020. https://www.statista.com/statistics/197569/annual-retail-and-food-services-sales/

2 Ingraham, C. "Lawns are a soul-crushing timesuck and most of us would be better off without them." The Washington Post. August 4, 2015. https://www.washingtonpost.com/news/wonk/wp/2015/08/04/lawns-are-a-soul-crushing-timesuck-and-most-of-us-would-be-better-off-without-them/

3 Holthaus, E. "Lawns are the No. 1 irrigated 'crop' in America. They need to die." Grist. May 2, 2019. https://grist.org/article/lawns-are-the-no-1-agricultural-crop-in-america-they-need-to-die/

4 Galhena, D.H., Freed, R., and Maredia, K.M. "Home gardens: a promising approach to enhance household food security and wellbeing." May 31, 2013. *BMC Agriculture & Food Security.* https://agricultureandfoodsecurity.biomedcentral.com/articles/10.1186/2048-7010-2-8

5 Cunningham, W.P. and Cunningham, M.A. *Environmental Science – A Global Concern.* 2018.

6 "Growing Better: Ten Critical Transitions to Transform Food and Land Use." The Food and Land Use Coalition. September, 2019. https://www.foodandlandusecoalition.org/global-report/

7 "Trucost reveals $3 trillion environmental cost of farming." *Trucost News.* October 15, 2015. https://www.trucost.com/trucost-news/trucost-reveals-3-trillion-environmental-cost-farming/

8   Tegymeier, E.M. and Duffy, M.D. "External costs
     of agricultural production in the United States".
     International Journal of Agricultural Sustainability.
     May 26, 2011. https://www.tandfonline.com/doi/
     abs/10.1080/14735903.2004.9684563
9   Hyman, M. *Food Fix – How to save our health, our economy,
     our communities, and our planet – one bite at a time.* Little,
     Brown, Spark. 2020.
10   Aspenson, A. "True" costs for food system reform:
     An overview of true cost accounting literature and
     initiatives. Johns Hopkins Center For A Livable Future.
     January 2020. https://clf.jhsph.edu/sites/default/
     files/2020-02/true-cost-for-food-system-reform-2020.
     pdf
11   Ibid
12   Kaplan, L. Energy (in)efficiency of the local food
     movement: food for thought. Fordham Environmental
     Law Review. Spring 2012. 23:139-161. https://www.jstor.
     org/stable/44175661?read-now=1&seq=1
13   DeVore, B. Counting calories in agriculture. Minnesota
     Environmental Partnership. November 10, 2006.
     https://www.mepartnership.org/counting-calories-in-
     agriculture/

Chapter 5

1   Solomon, St. *Gardening When it Counts.* 2005. New
     Society Publishers.

Chapter 6

1   Cotroneo, C. "Why the indoor farming movement is taking off." May 20, 2020. *Treehugger*. https://www. treehugger.com/indoor-farming-study-obstacles-growth-potential-4859467?utm_term=0_fcbff2e256-4b3a7b5f97-40239325&utm_campaign=4b3a7b5f97-RSS_EMAIL_CAMPAIGN_FRI0522_2020&utm_medium=email&utm_source=Weekly+Newsletter

2   Linnekin, B.J. *Biting the hand that feeds you*. 2016. Island Press.

Chapter 7

1   Solomon, St. *Gardening When it Counts*. 2005. New Society Publishers.

2   Ibid.

3   Danahy, A. "Purple power. 7 Benefits of purple potatoes." Nov. 20, 2019. *Healthline*. https://www.healthline.com/nutrition/purple-potatoes

4   Ibid.

5   Coleman, E. *Four-Season Harvest – Organic vegetables from your home garden all year long*. 1999. Chelsea Green Publishing Company.

Chapter 8

1   "Farms and land in farms. 2018 Summary." April 2019. USDA. https://www.nass.usda.gov/Publications/Todays_Reports/reports/fnlo0419.pdf

2   Merril, D. and Letherby, L. "Here's how America uses its land." July 31, 2018. Bloomberg. https://www.bloomberg.com/graphics/2018-us-land-use/

3   Francis Moore Lappe. *Diet for a small planet*. 1982. Ballantine Books.

4   "Does the United States import more agricultural products than we export?" Jan 11, 2021. American Farm Bureau Foundation for Agriculture. https:// www.agfoundation.org/common-questions/view/does-the-united-states-import-more-agricultural-products-than-we-export#:~:text=Agriculture%20has%20a%20 positive%20trade,and%20veggies%20topping%20the%20 list.

5   Meyer, K.S. "Which diet makes best use of farmland? You might be surprised." Ensia. July 22, 2016. https://ensia. com/notable/which-diet-makes-best-use-of-farmland-you-might-be-surprised/

6   Wuerthner, G. "The truth about land use in the United States." Summer, 2002. *Watersheds Messenger,* Vol. IX, no. 2. https://www.westernwatersheds.org/ watmess/watmess_2002/2002html_summer/article6. htm#:~:text=The%20amount%20of%20land%20 used,less%20than%203%20million%20acres

7   "Save the topsoil." Soil Solutions. October 16, 2018. https://soilsolutions.net/save-the-topsoil/

8   Lawton, K. "Economics of soil loss." *Farm Progress*. March 13, 2017. https://www.farmprogress.com/soil-health/ economics-soil-loss

9   Ibid.

10   Philpott, T. *Perilous bounty – The looming collapse of American farming and how we can prevent it*. 2020. Bloomsbury Publishing.

11   "Save the topsoil!" *Soil Solutions*. Oct. 16, 2018. https:// soilsolutions.net/save-the-topsoil/

12 USDA Economic Research Service. "Food security and nutrition assistance." Dec 16, 2020. https://www.ers.usda.gov/data-products/ag-and-food-statistics-charting-the-essentials/food-security-and-nutrition-assistance/#:~:text=In%202019%2C%2089.5%20percent%20of,than%202018%20(11.1%20percent).

13 Newby, P.K, Tucker, K.L., Wolk, A. "Risk of overweight and obesity among semivegetarian, lactovegetarian, and vegan women." American J. Clinical Nutrition 81:1267-74. June 2005. https://academic.oup.com/ajcn/article/81/6/1267/4648730

14 Wilson, D. "Eating meat is linked to obesity." Peta. https://www.peta.org/issues/animals-used-for-food/obesity/

15 Roland, J. "What's the average weight for men?" March 7,2019. *Healthline*. https://www.healthline.com/health/mens-health/average-weight-for-men#_noHeaderPrefixedContent

16 "Endoscopic weight loss program" Johns Hopkins Medicine. https://www.hopkinsmedicine.org/endoscopic-weight-loss-program/conditions/diabetes.html

17 Goldenbert, S. "Half of all US food produce is thrown away, new research suggests." July, 2016. *The Guardian*. https://www.theguardian.com/environment/2016/jul/13/us-food-waste-ugly-fruit-vegetables-perfect

18 "Supermarkets moving toward zero food waste." *Smart Sense*. Jan. 15,2020. https://blog.smartsense.co/supermarkets-zero-food-waste#:~:text=Supermarkets%20are%20responsible%20for%2010,and%20dairy%20products%20every%20year.

19 Pollack, H. "The USDA says Americans only eat three kinds of vegetables." Sept. 15, 2015. *Vice.* https://www. vice.com/en/article/vvxpy4/the-usda-says-americans-only-eat-three-kinds-of-vegetables

20 Nestle, M. "What fruits and vegetables do Americans eat? More charts from USDA." May 15, 2017. Menu. https://www.foodpolitics.com/2017/05/what-fruits-and-vegetables-do-americans-eat-more-charts-from-usda/

21 Renner, B. "Stunning survey reveals quarter of Americans have never eaten vegetables." Oct. 8, 2019. *Study Finds.* https://www.studyfinds.org/stunning-survey-reveals-1-in-4-adults-has-never-eaten-vegetables/#:~:text=Overall%2C%20a%20whopping%20 91.4%25%20of,%2Dliked%20vegetable%20at%2089%25.

Chapter 9

1 "Agriculture at a Crossroads – IAASTD Findings and Recommendations for Future Farming." Global report. UN Environment Programme. 2018. https://ali-sea.org/ aliseaonlinelibrary/agriculture-at-a-crossroads-iaastd-findings-and-recommendations-for-future-farming/

2 Ranganathan, J., Waite, R., Searchinger, T. and Hanson, C. "How to Sustainably Feed 10 Billion People by 2050, in 21 Charts." Dec. 5, 2018. World Resources Institute. https://www.wri.org/blog/2018/12/how-sustainably-feed-10-billion-people-2050-21-charts

3 *Growing Better report 2019.* The Food and Land Use Coalition. https://www.foodandlandusecoalition.org/ global-report/

4   "World Economic Forum's 'Great Reset' Plan for Big
     Food Benefits Industry, Not People." *The Defender.* Nov.
     9, 2020. https://childrenshealthdefense.org/defender/
     world-economic-forums-great-reset-plan-for-big-food-
     benefits-industry-not-people/

5   Galhena, D.H., Freed, R., and Maredia, K.M. "Home
     Gardens: a Promising Approach to Enhance
     Household Food Security and Wellbeing." *BMC
     Agriculture & Food Security.* May 31, 2013. https://
     agricultureandfoodsecurity.biomedcentral.com/
     articles/10.1186/2048-7010-2-8

6   Philpott, T. *Perilous bounty – The looming collapse of
     American farming and how we can prevent it.* 2020.
     Bloomsbury Publishing.

7   "U.S. Food Retail Industry – Statistics and Facts." Nov. 5,
     2020. *Stastista.* https://www.statista.com/topics/1660/
     food-retail/#dossierSummary__chapter1

8   Philpott, T. *Perilous bounty – The looming collapse of
     American farming and how we can prevent it.*2020.
     Bloomsbury Publishing.

9   "Scotts Miracle-Gro shares uptick of gardening statistics
     related to COVID-19." *Garden Center.* June 8, 2020.
     https://www.gardencentermag.com/article/scotts-
     miracle-gro-shares-gardening-statistics-covid-19/

Appendix 1

1   Foley, J. "It's time to rethink America's corn system."
     Scientific American. March 5, 2013. https://www.
     scientificamerican.com/article/time-to-rethink-corn/

Appendix 2

1   "Fertilizing with human urine." Veganic Agriculture
    Network. https://goveganic.net/article217.html
2   Krueger, S. How much nitrogen does your corn need?
    Emergence. June 17, 2018. https://emergence.fbn.com/
    agronomy/how-much-nitrogen-does-your-corn-need
3   "Nitrogen fertilization of corn." Penn State Extension.
    February 11, 2005. https://extension.psu.edu/nitrogen-
    fertilization-of-corn
4   Foley, J. "It's time to rethink America's corn system."
    Scientific American. March 5, 2013. https://www.
    scientificamerican.com/article/time-to-rething-corn/
5   Cunningham, W.P. and Cunningham, M.A.
    Environmental Science – A Global Concern. 2018.